# RECIPES

—BY—

# LADIES OF ST. PAUL'S

# RECIPES

—BY—

# LADIES OF ST. PAUL'S

P. E. CHURCH,

AKRON, OHIO.

---

COMPILED BY

MISS HARRIET ANGEL.

---

A NEW EDITION WITH A PHOTO INSERT AND
AN INTRODUCTION BY JON MILLER

BUCHTEL BOOKS • AKRON, OHIO

Originally published 1887 by The Werner Printing and Manufacturing Company



13 12 11 10 09 5 4 3 2 1

ISBN 978-1-931968-67-6

The paper used in this publication meets the minimum requirements of American National Standard for Information Sciences—Permanence of Paper for Printed Library Materials, ANSI Z39.48–1984. ∞

Cover image: St. Paul's, circa 1890s. Courtesy of Archival Services, University Libraries, The University of Akron.

Cover design: Amy Freels

DEDICATED TO

MRS. FRANK ADAMS,

President Ladies' Aid Society,
St. Paul's P. E. Church.

# INDEX.

# PREFACE TO THE ORIGINAL EDITION

We may live without poetry, music, or art;
We may live without conscience, live without heart;
We may live without friends; may live without books;
But civilized men cannot live without cooks.

and, though it is asserted that, like poets, cooks are born, not made, good cooking is largely the result of practical experience.

It is the truest economy to concoct the given materials into dishes so palatable and so daintily served that waste shall be reduced to a minimum. Since, "in the multitude of councilors there is wisdom," may we be pardoned if we add another to the number of cook books already flooding the land, as all the formulae given in this compilation are obtained from ladies whose dainties are acknowledged to be most toothsome, and who, by this method, furnish the recipes for which they have often been importuned. The editors were troubled with *un embarras des riches*, and, perhaps the selections are not the most felictitous, but "to err is human." We tender our sincere thanks to the ladies of our town, and especially to those of other congregations who have responded to our requests generously.

EDITORIAL COMMITTEE.

*Akron, Ohio, April 12, 1887.*

# INTRODUCTION
## Jon Miller

Between 1880 and 1890, the City of Akron grew from about 10,000 people to about 28,000 people. Akron would not enter the list of America's 100 most populated cities until the 1900 census, but in 1887 it was undoubtedly an urban area with a thriving industrial center. The city produced cereals, clay products, sewer pipes, and rubber goods that were easily and profitably shipped to other markets through the city's canals and railroads.

### GETTING AND PREPARING FOOD IN 1887 AKRON

By 1887, Akron families no longer lived in log cabins; one and two-story wood-frame houses were common. Public utilities were becoming more readily available, and the citizens of Akron were making a gradual transition to life with running water and natural gas. Water is essential for cooking, of course, and water quality was a key consideration when preparing meals in that era. Before the advent of city water and sewers, people depended on springs, wells, and cisterns. Spring and well water had to be carried into the house. Cisterns were brick or cement structures built into the ground and filled by downspouts collecting rainwater from the roof. A typical cistern held about 100 gallons of water; it required a filtration system (usually stone), and it had to be cleaned often. Hot water for cleaning, laundry, and bathing was not supplied by a hot-water heater but by a pot that lived on the kitchen stove.

Arthur H. Blower remembered his childhood in 1885–1900 Akron in a 1955 book published by the Summit County Historical Society. Without gas, Akron families lit their homes with kerosene lamps, and they burned coal or wood in the kitchen stove. The introduction of gas horrified many citizens of Akron in the late 1880s and 1890s, Blower writes, because they were sure "it would explode in our stoves and blow us to Kingdom Come."

Homeowners typically purchased gas for improved interior lighting, but a home that was piped for natural gas would soon have a gas stove in the kitchen. Coal and wood stoves required constant attention to maintain a good fire. Gas stoves provided quick heat for boiling, baking, roasting, or frying and were regarded as a great convenience for the housekeeper. The gas stove was much cleaner as well, and in the summer gas stoves were greatly admired for not overheating both the kitchen and the whole house. "A dinner can be cooked with gas in a white dress, and the mistress can appear perfectly cool and bearing none but savory reminders of her hour in the kitchen," wrote one author for a woman's magazine of the day.

There were drawbacks to gas stoves, however. Most homes still required extended burning hours of a coal or wood stove for heat in the winter and for the availability of hot water to meet the demands of the family. Therefore, when first introduced, the gas stove only supplemented the coal or wood stove, and it was regarded by some as an unnecessary new-fangled invention. Gas stoves could also burn at startlingly high temperatures. Many housekeepers initially scorched the meals that cooked longer and at lower temperatures in a coal or wood stove.

Over time, however, the coal or wood stove disappeared from the kitchen and the gas stove came to be regarded as efficient, superior, and essential. Though he regretted "that the cheerfulness of a coal or a wood fire" was "gone forever from our kitchens," Arthur Blower remembered that the introduction of natural gas was a "blessing for mothers in the kitchen."

Electricity also came to the city in the 1880s. Electricity was not immediately useful in the home; at the time gas lighting was superior to electric lighting. Businesses used enormous electric lights that they erected on the corners of Akron's downtown streets to promote their operations. At first, the lights were a marvel; they attracted people to the business district like moths to a flame. Electricity had other early uses. In 1888, the first electric streetcar ran down Market Street.

With electricity came the telephone. Like electricity, the telephone was much more appealing to businesses than to private homes, and it became an essential tool for doing business. If a store had a phone, the proprietor could answer questions about the quality and availability of products prior to delivery. Ten advertisements in this cookbook include telephone numbers—three-digit phone numbers for architects, purveyors of fine furniture in "chaste designs," sellers of meat, wall paper, and groceries. The telephone was also used to arrange for coal delivery, gas fittings, plumbing service, and mortuary service.

The 1880s were "the horse and buggy days" of Akron; getting around town to shop for essentials was not pleasant or easy. An Akron circus performer named Achille "Archie" Phillion began construction of his "steam carriage," a primitive early automobile, around 1887. But he did not drive his unreliable spectacle until the early 1890s, when bicycles were gaining in popularity in Akron and across the country. (Akron's rubber manufacturers thrived on the production and sale of bicycle tires.) The city's roads were not wide and smooth, and few were paved. Since transportation was dependent on horses and mules, Akron had plenty of stables, livery barns, feed stores, harness shops, hay markets, wagon-repair shops, carriage factories, and manure piles. When streetcars were first introduced in the early 1880s, they were powered not by electricity but by horses and mules. By city ordinance, the new mode of conveyance was limited to speeds of five miles per hour or less.

Since travel within the city was slow and dirty, most food was delivered to the house. Milk peddlers travelled daily routes in small, lightweight wagons with a canvas top. The sellers rang bells as they moved down a street. People grabbed their pitchers and jugs and went to the wagon to buy milk by the pint or the quart. Fish peddlers came less often, maybe once a week, tooting horns in a signature fashion and selling strings of scaled, deboned, and beheaded fish. Fish would not keep, so an Akron household would need recipes for leftovers from a fish dinner.

During the era, Americans were interested in finding a way to improve their means of artificial refrigeration, mainly to meet the demands of the brewing industries and the need for well-refrigerated railroad cars. In the 1880s, "refrigeration" in a private home meant keeping the windows open, using a gas stove in the summer, and maintaining a messy icebox, which cooled a small space in a rather unreliable fashion.

Processed or canned food was not a household staple until the early 1900s, around the time Upton Sinclair wrote *The Jungle* (1906). But in the late 1800s, Akron was home to Ferdinand Schumacher, the German immigrant, Prohibition Party politician, and "Oatmeal King" of America. His method of processing oats created a widespread demand for the cereal. After several mergers, Schumacher's cereal companies eventually became the Quaker Oats Company.

Akron housekeepers of the late 19th century mainly prepared fresh foods or foods that had longer shelf lives like winter potatoes. Local farmers brought their seasonal products into town for sale in groceries and by peddlers, who sold farm produce, such as potatoes and watermelon, from horse-drawn wagons. Arthur Blower remembered that these "hucksters" distinguished themselves not with bells or horns but with the musical bellowing of their product—*PO–TA–A–TO–O–E–S* or *WADDY–MELO–O–O–ONS*—much like beer vendors now do at baseball games.

With better roads and the rise of streetcars, groceries grew and were always busy on Saturday nights. Most people worked a sixty-hour week, and Saturday night was a common time off to come to town under the electric lights. Men collected in the grocery stores to loaf, gossip, and perhaps to haggle for perishable goods before the Sunday closing. New roads allowed Akron's F. W. Albrecht to expand his grocery business from the one store he opened at the corner of Buchtel Avenue and Center Street in 1891. By 1904, his chain of "Acme" stores grew to six since he was able to dependably and cheaply deliver goods from a central warehouse to small residential groceries that, in turn, delivered food to Akron homes. In 1916 the Acme stores stopped delivery and became "basket" stores. Customers then had to travel to the store, select and purchase their groceries, and transport them home themselves.

The ingredients in these recipes include the staple items for citizens of Akron in 1887. They ate a lot of potatoes, they made a lot of soup with perishable produce, and they found ways to mix and fry up scraps of leftover meat and fish. If the recipes seem heavy or calorie-rich by today's standards, note that Americans of the late 1800s struggled to meet their energy needs. Unlike today, when the average American can easily consume far more calories than he or she needs on a daily basis, in the 19th century the opposite was true. The heaviness of these foods testifies not to their gluttony but to their struggle to get the calories they needed. Undoubtedly, some of the city's wealthiest citizens were rather well-fed, however, and may have enjoyed the face that obesity was generally respected as a display of wealth during the era.

## RECIPES BY LADIES OF ST. PAUL'S PROTESTANT EPISCOPAL CHURCH

St. Paul's Episcopal Church was organized in 1836, meeting at various places, including the old "Stone Block" at the corner of Howard and Market Streets. In 1844 the church settled in a wood-frame building on South High Street before moving, in 1885, to the stone building on the western corner of East Market and Forge. The larger stone building, west of the original church building, was added in 1907. The current church on West Market Street was consecrated in 1952.

The 1885 building is just one reason The Reverend Leo Ganter is remembered as one of St. Paul's most successful rectors. Built on what would be known as the versatile "Akron plan" of church architecture, St. Paul's had a large worship space that opened into a series of smaller cubicle rooms around its perimeter. The smaller rooms had many uses and were used, for example, for Sunday School classes during the worship service.

The Sunday School was a busy one. In 1887, St. Paul's had about 330 church members and an equal number of Sunday School students. The congregation appears to have been made up of large, young families, and the church enjoyed a bustling social life. The church archives include evidence of a wide variety of social events, and these events often involved a large part of the entire congregation. Handwritten programs for the annual church picnics of 1887 and 1888, for example, show that about half the adult congregation were given vital assignments on the required committees for "transportation," "tables," "waiters," "lemonade," and so forth. These picnic programs also include nearly all of the names signed to recipes in this cookbook.

*Recipes by Ladies of St. Paul's P.E. Church* documents more than the dietary tastes and habits of the time. It also demonstrates the organizational skills of the women involved. As Kathleen L. Endres has shown in her book, *Akron's Better Half: Women's Clubs and the Humanization of the City, 1825–1925*, the city was thoroughly organized by women who were interested in escaping the kitchen stove and somehow contributing to improvements in the quality of life for all of Akron's citizens. St. Paul's Episcopal Church was no different than Akron's other churches in this regard: the women organized for a variety of causes. This cookbook may have been created and marketed for some specific charitable cause. If not, the proceeds surely went, eventually, to the support of the charitable work of St. Paul's generous and organized women. At St. Paul's, the women were especially interested in helping the children of Akron. Calling themselves "The Heart and Hand Circle of St. Paul's Episcopal Church," women of St. Paul's ran a chapter of The Order of the King's Daughters, an international women's organization; in 1890 they worked with another Protestant chapter of the King's Daughters in Akron to found a day nursery for the children of Akron's working women, which grew into Akron Children's Hospital.

The cookbook includes contributions from a founder of this woman's circle, Mary Folger Rawson Perkins, the wife of George Tod Perkins, who signed her "salmon salad" and "dressing for sandwiches" with the name, "Mrs. G. T. Perkins." In 1890, her daughter Mary wed a son of another long-established Akron family, Charles B. Raymond. Then a rubber-industry secretary, Raymond would eventually serve as an important executive at B. F. Goodrich. Certainly, she married more than a man—she married a family with culinary traditions that evidently included, in this case, "whortleberry pudding," "fricassed oysters," and "Annie's lemon pie."

Other notable contributions to this cookbook are signed with the name of Colonel A. L. Conger, whose postwar experience as a travelling salesman of farm machinery led to the presidency of the enormously successful Whitman & Barnes Manufacturing Company. On the side he served as the President of the Akron Steam Forge Company, a director of the Second National Bank of Akron, the Chairman of the Summit County Republican Committee, and he had a large interest in local straw, building, lumber, plate glass, tin plate, and railway companies. At home "Mrs. A. L. Conger," Emily Bronson Conger, prepared (or oversaw the preparation of) "orange sherbet," "pineapple sherbet," and "apple cream."

Other names are easily recognized as associated with notable citizens of nineteenth-century Akron. One frequent contributor here is "Mrs. D. L. King," who surely is the wife of David Leicester King, who graduated from Harvard College in 1846 and moved to Akron in 1849 to practice law with his brother as "King & King." King left law and became secretary of the Akron Sewer Pipe Company. When this cookbook was published, he was President of the King Varnish Company and the Glendale Cemetary Company. His wife, Bettie Washington Steele King, was a grandniece of George Washington. She served "bean soup," "tomato soup," "potato soup," "celery soup," "baked fish," "sweetbread salad," "lemon pudding," "gelatine pudding," and a "corn starch cocoanut pudding." Her daughter, "Miss King," was expert in preparing "salad dressing" and "pudding sauce."

The cookbook not only tells us what these people ate, but it also says a great deal about the way the people of Akron were connected to one another. The advertisements had to be sold; someone from St. Paul's walked down East Market Street and up and down Howard and Main, and thus commanded dozens of advertisement purchases.

A church member went to Cleveland, evidently on the train, and sold ad space to store owners on Euclid Avenue. (Also on Euclid Avenue was St. Paul's Episcopal Church of Cleveland.)

Finally, the recipes in the cookbook are worth trying today. The ladies of St. Paul did not record recipes in the "scientific" fashion of the twentieth century. Though some surely prepared these recipes with a gas stove, nearly all that involved heat for baking, roasting, stewing, etc. were invented and perfected on a coal or wood stove. These stoves were not precisely regulated as present-day stoves, and therefore, these recipes do not specify the actual oven temperature. For most purposes, a 350 degree oven should be fine. As for measures, experimentation with the amounts of ingredients might be necessary to get good results. That said, most of the recipes are not complicated, and even an amateur cook could recreate them by practice and consulting modern recipes for similar creations.

Bon appetit.

# BIBLIOGRAPHY


Blower, Arthur H. *Akron at the Turn of the Century, 1890–1913*. Akron: Summit County Historical Society, 1955.

"Cooking with Gas." *Christian Union* 38.22 (November 29, 1888) 611.

Endres, Kathleen H. *Akron's "Better Half": Women's Clubs and the Humanization of the City, 1825–1925*. Akron: University of Akron Press, 2006.

Jackson, James S. and Margot Y. Jackson. *At Home on the Hill: The Perkins Family of Akron*. Akron: Summit County Historical Society, 1983.

Lane, Samuel A. *Fifty Years and Over of Akron and Summit County*. 1892. Barberton, Ohio: Barberton Historical Society, 1979.

McClain, Shirla Robinson. *The Contributions of Blacks in Akron: 1825–1975*. Edited by The Akron Gallery of Black History Curriculum Committee. Akron: The University of Akron, 1996.

McGovern, Frances. *Written on the Hills: The Making of the Akron Landscape*. Updated ed. Akron: Univeristy of Akron Press, 1996.

Olin, Oscar Eugene, et al, editors. *A Centennial History of Akron, 1825–1925*. Akron: Summit County Historical Society, 1925.

Olin, Oscar Eugene. *Akron and Environs: Historical, Biographical, Genealogical*. Chicago and New York: Lewis, 1917.

# RECIPES

—BY—

# LADIES OF ST. PAUL'S

## P. E. CHURCH,

## AKRON, OHIO.

---

COMPILED BY

MISS HARRIET ANGEL.

**SYNONYMS** 25,000 Words in ordinary use. Very accurate, neat and attractive. Price, by mail, 10 cents.

**Words Correctly Spoken,** by Elroy M. Avery, Ph. D. Wittily written. Beautifully printed with red-line borders; bound in cloth. Price, by mail, 15c. These books copyrighted and published by THE BURROWS BROS. CO., Publishers, Booksellers and Stationers Cleveland, O. Ask your bookseller for these books, and make him keep them.

## TO THE LADIES OF ST. PAUL'S.

*Dear Mesdames:*—With the hope that our action may assist you in the sale of your Cook Book, we hereby agree to accept copies of the same in place of money to the full amount of the list price on purchases from our retail stock, to the amount of ten dollars or over; one copy only to be accepted at a time, and this offer to hold good during the year 1887. Trusting that this may be a help to you in disposing of them freely, and hoping your fair may be otherwise successful, we are,

Yours Very Respectfully,

**THE BURROWS BROS. CO.,**

23, 25 & 27 Euclid Avenue, CLEVELAND, OHIO.

**SYNONYMS** 25,000 Words in ordinary use. Very accurate, neat and attractive. Price, by mail 10 cents.

**Words Correctly Spoken,** by Elroy M. Avery, Ph. D. Wittily written. Beautifully printed with red-line borders; bound in cloth. Price, by mail 15c. These books copyrighted and published by THE BURROWS BROS. CO., publishers, booksellers and stationers Cleveland, O. Ask your bookseller for these books, and make him keep them.

The LARGEST STORE and the Largest Stock of

# Books and Stationery

In the State of Ohio, and outside of Chicago, in the west, is that of

## THE BURROWS BROS. CO.,

23, 25 & 27 Euclid Avenue,

CLEVELAND, O.

To spend several days in a friend's house and hunger for something to read while you are treading on costly carpets, sitting upon luxurious chairs, and sleeping under coverlids of eider, is—how forlorn, and, alas, how common! Given a taste for reading and the means of gratifying it, and you can hardly fail to make a happy man. Why not, therefore, if you have children, cultivate in them a taste which will stand by them in every variety of circumstances, a taste which, if not acquired before the age of maturity, will come after that with difficulty. Are you in moderate circumstances? Remember that books, the reading of them, and the knowledge that comes from the study of books, are what distinguish the highest civilization with its comfort-giving appliances from the lowest barbarism and its attendant squalor. Are you, on the contrary, in possession of wealth enough to insure you comforts and luxuries? Then remember, that NO HOUSE IS FURNISHED UNTIL IT HAS BOOKS AND A LIBRARY. Why spend hundreds and thousands of dollars on carpets, curtains and bric-a-brac more freely than tens for books? "It is books that teach us to refine our pleasures when young, and having so taught us, enable us to recall them with satisfaction when old," we are told by Leigh Hunt. Nearly all knowledge is useful to the man who would be broad-minded. An acquaintance with chemistry may be of more value to a preacher than he would ever deem possible; military tactics may not be without value to a publisher, as witness the notable English house of John Murray, and the essence of the doctrine of evolution may preserve an architect for abiding in the time-worn ruts of the past. The invention of Henry Bessemer of converting steel, which made its author twenty-five millions and the world one hundred millions of profits or savings, was that of a broadly enlightened man, not an iron worker, who turned all the force of his brain power to that subject. "Qui legit regit," said the old Romans, and the commentaries of perhaps the most remarkable man who has ever lived on this earth will go far to prove the assertion true. "Arbor scientæ, arbor vitæ," is the motto chosen by that sweetest of English poets, Austin Dobson, for the title-page of one of his books. Therefore, we say again:

**BUY BOOKS!**

**BUY THEM OF US IF YOU WILL.**

**BUT BUY THEM.**

OUR BLOCK is now being remodeled. When ready for business, about June first, we give you all a cordial invitation to visit us and inspect our establishment. In the meantime, while we are torn up and in uninviting shape, we will do the best we are able to give your orders our prompt attention.

**The Burrows Bros. Co.**

**SYNONYMS** 25,000 Words in ordinary use. Very accurate, neat and attractive. price, by mail 10 cents

**Words Correctly Spoken,** by Elroy M. Avery, Ph. D. Wittily written. Beautifully printed with red-line borders; bound in cloth. price, by mail 15c. These books copyrighted and published by THE BURROWS BROS. CO., publishers, booksellers and stationers Cleveland, O. Ask your bookseller for these books, and make him keep them.

"Without books, God is silent, justice dormant, natural science at a stand, philosophy lame, letters dumb and all things involved in Cimmerian darkness."—*Bartholin.*

"It is a man's duty to have books. A library is not a luxury, but one of the necessaries of a right life.—*Henry Ward Beecher.*"

**WITH LOW PRICES AND BEST GOODS**

We hope to merit your trade and convince you that the old Norman-French motto, which we have chosen to copy from one of the poets, as the legend of our escutcheon is deserved: **"Autant Icy Qu'ailleurs."**

**SYNONYMS** 25,000 Words in ordinary use. Very accurate, neat and attractive. Price, by mail, 10 cents.

**Words Correctly Spoken,** by Elroy M. Avery, Ph. D. Wittily written. Beautifully printed with red-line borders; bound in cloth. Price, by mail, 15c. These books copyrighted and published by THE BURROWS BROS. CO., Publishers, Booksellers and Stationers Cleveland, O. Ask your bookseller for these books, and make him keep them.

# DELICATESSE

—FROM OUR—

# CUISINE DELICATE

In the Front Window at the

# PHILADELPHIA * DAIRY * AND * CAFE,

69 EUCLID AVENUE,

## CLEVELAND, - OHIO.

---

THIS Homelike and Unique Hostelry is conducted on the European Plan; is open Day and Nigh., is brilliantly illuminated with Incandescent Electric Lights. It is unquestionably the *most popular resort* in Cleveland.

---

## ICE CREAM, OYSTERS, LUNCHEON OR MEALS

ARE SERVED AT ALL HOURS.

---

IT has an **Elegant Ladies' Parlor,** cosy, and entirely secluded. It has the

## LARGEST LADIES' PATRONAGE

OF ANY HOUSE IN CLEVELAND.

---

**It is First-Class in all its Appointments.**

ENTRANCE AT

## 69 EUCLID AVENUE,

**Opp. the Opera House, CLEVELAND, O.**

# Barrett's Music Emporium

**92 Euclid Avenue, CLEVELAND, OHIO.**

**LARGE STOCK,**
**ELEGANT STYLES,**

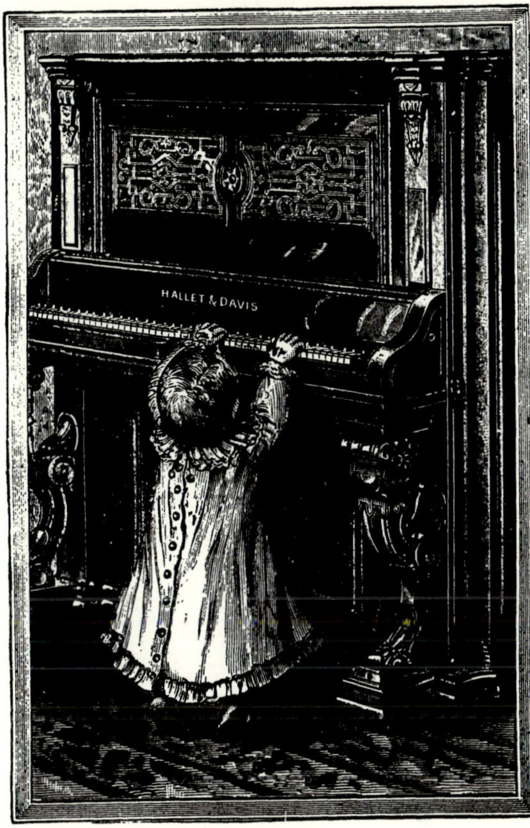


**TERMS EASY,**
**PRICES RIGHT.**

Every Piano that we handle, however plain the casing may be, has the very best interior work, showing that great pains has been taken by the maker, and is built for a life time of service.

—REPRESENTED BY—

## W. K. RANDALL,

**ARCADE BLOCK - - - AKRON, OHIO.**

# RECIPES.

## SOUPS.

"Hail Soup! thou harbinger of a good dinner."
"Good diet, with wisdom, best comfort man."

*Bean Soup.*—Soak one quart black beans over night. In the morning, put on to boil with three pounds beef and a small piece of pork, one head of celery, two grated carrots. Boil two hours, seasoning to taste with salt, pepper, cloves, allspice and cinnamon. Strain through the colander, and put into a tureen in which has been placed two hard boiled eggs, sliced, one lemon sliced and one teaspoonful tomato catsup. Mrs. D. L. King.

*Tomato Soup.*—Boil together until done one quart tomatoes, one and one-half pint water, two small potatoes, one onion, or none, strain through a colander, add pepper, salt, butter and one teacup hot milk with a trifle corn starch stirred in. Miss Carpenter.

*Tomato Soup.*—Boil together, one can tomatoes, three pints water, one onion, one tablespoonful of butter, season with salt and pepper, and strain through a colander and add one pint milk, or cream, boiled and thickened with a little rolled cracker. Serve at once. Mrs. D. L. King.

*Green Pea Soup.*—Boil one can green peas in one quart of water and a little onion for twenty minutes. Add one quart of milk, and one tablespoonful melted butter, two of flour with enough of the soup to make a smooth, thin mixture worked thoroughly together, added to the soup, boil ten minutes, season with salt and pepper and strain. Mrs. N. P. Goodhue.

*Potato Soup.*—Boil four medium sized potatoes in water till soft, mash fine and strain through a soup strainer. At same time boil milk with a small onion long enough to flavor. Just before serving, put strained potatoes into milk with tablespoonful butter and a little salt. Mrs. D. L. King.

*Corn Soup.*—Boil in one quart of water, till well done, one dozen ears of corn, cut and scraped, then add two quarts sweet milk, bring to a boil, then add one-fourth pound butter, smoothed into two tablespoonfuls flour, season with salt and pepper. Pour the boiling soup over the well beaten yolks of two eggs, stirring constantly.

---

*Celery Soup.*—Boil two heads of celery in a pint of water thirty or forty minutes. At the same time boil together a pint of milk, a slice of onion and a small piece of mace, adding a tablespoonful butter and a tablespoonful of flour after it has boiled ten minutes. Mash the celery in the water in which it has been boiled and stir into the milk, season with salt and pepper and serve immediately. Fry little pieces of bread in hot lard and add when the soup has been put in the tureen. A cup of whipped cream improves this dish. Mrs. D. L. King.

---

*Chicken Soup.*—To the broth in which chickens have been boiled for salad, &c., add one onion, eight tomatoes, season with pepper and salt, boil thirty minutes. Just before serving stir in the well beaten yolks of two eggs.

---

*Noodles for Soup.*—Add to one egg as much sifted flour as it will absorb, with a little salt. Roll this as thin as a wafer, dredge very lightly with flour, and roll over into a roll. Slice off thinly from the ends, shake the strips out loosely, put into the soup, and serve with it. Mrs. J. A. M.

# SOUTH ❋ END ❋ GALLERY,

**A. L. HUBBARD, Operator.**

**Corner Middlebury and South Main Streets, AKRON, O.**

---

Photographic work of all descriptions done neatly and promptly.

*Remember we make CHILDRENS' PHOTOS a Specialty.*

**Outdoor work of any size and descrtption done at a moments' notice.**

---

ORDER YOUR MEATS OF

# A. KATZENBERG,

# California Meat Market,

**222 East Market Street, AKRON, OHIO.**

TELEPHONE, 139.

---

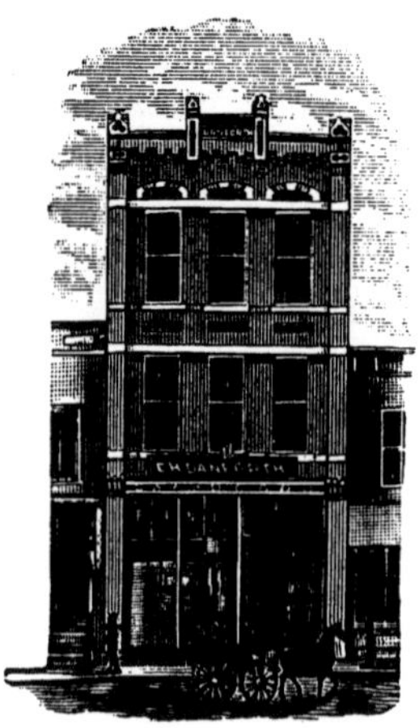

## E. H. DANFORTH,

# Wall Paper,

Oil Cloths and Window Shades,

**PAINTS, OILS, VARNISHES, BRUSHES, &c.**

---

**Art Decorations a Specialty.**

---

**309 Mill Street, - AKRON, O.**

TELEPHONE, NO. 396.

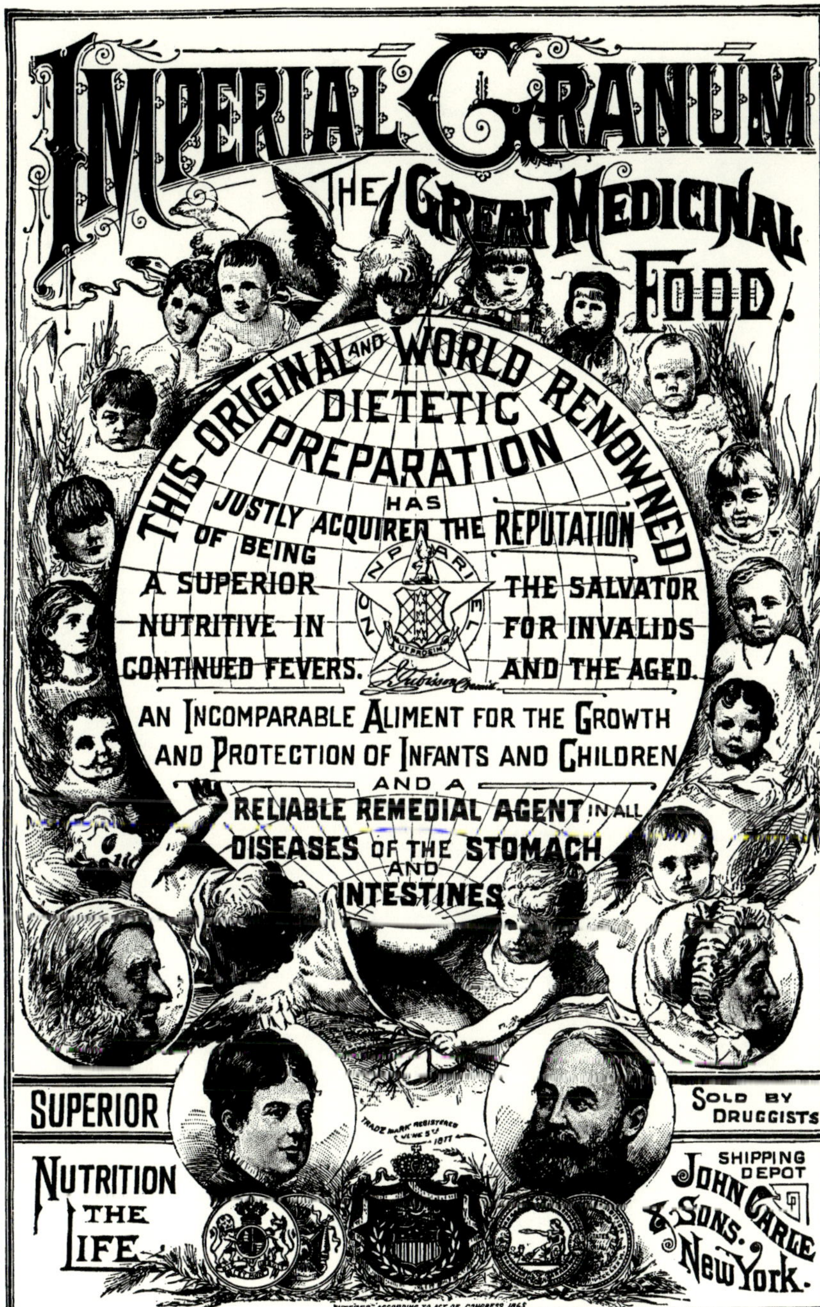
IMPERIAL GRANUM
THE GREAT MEDICINAL FOOD.
THIS ORIGINAL AND WORLD RENOWNED
DIETETIC PREPARATION
HAS JUSTLY ACQUIRED THE REPUTATION OF BEING
A SUPERIOR NUTRITIVE IN CONTINUED FEVERS.
THE SALVATOR FOR INVALIDS AND THE AGED.
NONPAREIL
AN INCOMPARABLE ALIMENT FOR THE GROWTH AND PROTECTION OF INFANTS AND CHILDREN
AND A
RELIABLE REMEDIAL AGENT IN ALL DISEASES OF THE STOMACH AND INTESTINES
SUPERIOR
NUTRITION THE LIFE
SOLD BY DRUGGISTS
SHIPPING DEPOT
JOHN CARLE & SONS. NEW YORK.
ENTERED ACCORDING TO ACT OF CONGRESS 1865

# CARRIAGES.

---

If you need anything in our line, we respectfully invite you to call and look through our stock, and get our prices.

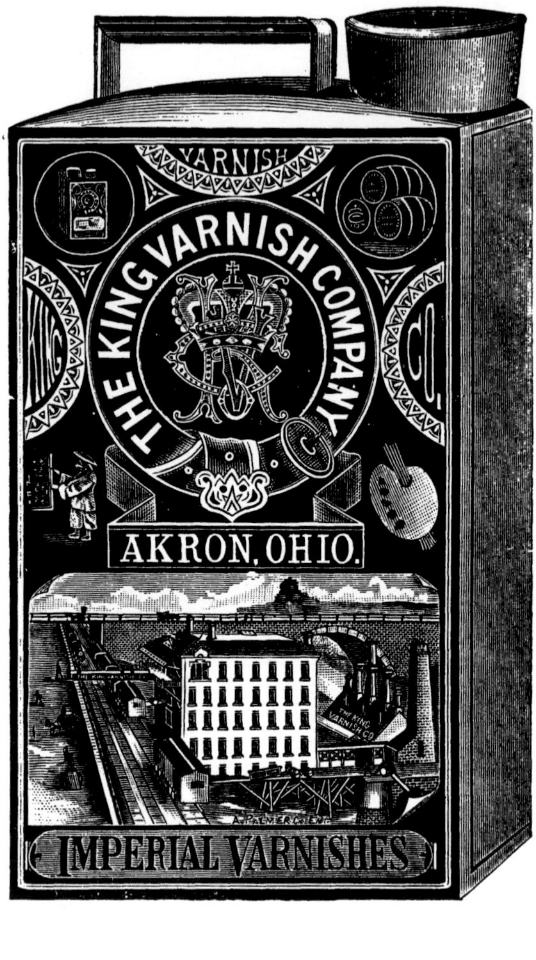
VARNISH
THE KING VARNISH COMPANY
KING
CO.
AKRON, OHIO.
THE KING VARNISH CO.
IMPERIAL VARNISHES

# FISH.

"Not all on hooks their criticism waste;
The genius of a dish some justly taste,
And eat their way to fame."

*Baked White Fish.*—Clean the fish and rub salt over it; make a stuffing of bread crumbs seasoned with salt, pepper and a little sage. Fill the fish, tie it up and bake. Any other than white fish may be used.

Or this method may be used: Clean the fish nicely, salt to taste, and lay it out flat (the back being cut nearly through) in a greased dripping pan, the flesh side laid up. Scatter pieces of butter on the fish and bake till done, from twenty minutes to half on hour, according to the size of the fish. When done pour over the fish a cupful of sweet cream and return to the oven till browned. A very hot oven is required to cook a fish in this way.

---

*Baked Blue Fish.*—Clean thoroughly, rub well, inside and out, with salt and pepper, dredge well with flour, place in a dripping pan with enough water to prevent scorching, add to the water a good sized lump of butter, and baste often. Miss Lansing.

---

*Baked Fish.*—Wash thoroughly, wipe dry, and fill with dressing of bread crumbs to which a little minced onion, chopped parsley, butter, pepper and salt have been added. Bind the fish by winding a cord several times around it, that the stuffing may not fall out, lay over the top a few strips of pork, sprinkle with salt and pepper, put some hot water in the pan and baste very often.

The following is a fine dressing for the fish: Put a small piece of butter into a sauce pan, when hot stir in a tablespoonful of flour, letting it remain till thoroughly cooked. Then add a teacup of boiling water, when boiling, take from the fire, add the yolks of four well beaten eggs, return to the fire a moment, to set the eggs, but not to boil, stir in juice of half a lemon, and a little more butter. Mrs. D. L. King.

---

*Codfish Balls.*—One-half pint of codfish, one pint of potatoes chopped fine, one egg, butter half size of an egg and a little pepper. Pick the fish very fine, put the potatoes in the fish-boiler to boil with the fish on top, cover with boiling water and cook for half an hour, drain, mash together till fine and light, add butter, pepper and egg, well beaten, drop into hot lard and cook brown. The spoon should be dipped into the hot lard before taking each spoonful of batter. Mrs. C. A. Collins.

---

*Broiled Cod Fish.*—Soak the codfish over night in plenty of luke-warm water. In the morning dry and broil on a well greased gridiron till nicely browned. When on the platter, add butter and pepper. Miss Francis.

---

*Fish a la Creme.*—Cook four pounds white fish in salted water with one tablespoonful of vinegar, until the flesh separates easily. Drain, and when cool remove the skin and bones. Pick apart in flakes and sprinkle with salt and pepper. Arrange on a platter (the same one in which you serve) first a layer of fish, then the dressing, then fish, repeating till all the fish is used, the top being dressing upon which one cup of rolled cracker, moistened with one-half cup melted butter, are spread. Set the platter in the oven, over a pan of hot water (to prevent cracking), and bake till crumbs are brown. It will need one pint of white sauce, made from this recipe: Heat two tablespoonfuls of butter and stir in two tablespoonfuls of flour, add carefully one pint of milk, stirring until perfectly smooth, then take from the fire and add one-half tablespoonful salt, same quantity onion juice, one-half salt spoonful pepper, one tablespoonful chopped parsley and same quantity of lemon juice. Mrs. W. C. Jacobs.

---

*Boiled Canned Salmon.*—Remove the paper wrapping of the can. Punch holes into each end of the can and put into a kettle of boiling water and boil it thirty minutes. Turn the salmon into a dish and serve with drawn butter and hard boiled eggs.

Miss Francis.

---

*Codfish Balls.*—Boil together, till well done, one-third codfish, picked very fine, and two-thirds raw potatoes cut into small dice; mash thoroughly, add butter and enough milk to moisten, mold into small cakes, fry in boiling lard, sufficient to cover them. If the fish be very salt, boil up once before adding the potatoes.

Mrs. J. A. Mason.

---

*Codfish Balls.*—One cup of codfish, one pint of potatoes, one teaspoonful of butter, one teaspoonful of flour, one egg well beaten, salt and pepper to taste.

Cut the potatoes into quarters, shred the fish, and boil both together until tender, (always put the fish on top of the potatoes,) drain and mash until the potatoes cannot be distingushed from the fish, then add seasoning and the egg. Put this mixture, by the spoonful, into a frying basket and immerse it into smoking hot fat, letting it cook a minute, or until browned. Drain on brown paper. Use leaf lard as for frying doughnuts The test for fat when frying fish balls, is to brown a piece of bread in it while counting forty.

---

*Sauce for Fish Balls.*—Two teaspoonfuls of salt, one teaspoonful each of flour, sugar and butter, two teaspoonfuls vinegar, one-half cup boiling water. Mrs. Fred. Ely, Cleveland.

---

*Clam or Fish Chowder.*—Put a few slices of salt pork into an iron kettle and fry until crisp; remove the pieces and chop them fine and put in a layer of fish or clams, then a layer of split crackers and potatoes, then another layer of fish, repeating till all is used, mixing in the chopped pork with salt pepper and minced onions, pour over boiling water, cover closely and stew till the fish is done. Mrs. P. W. Leavitt.

---

*Oyster Patties.*—Set one quart of oysters, with enough liquor to cover them, on the stove in a sauce pan, let them come to a boil, skim well, add two tablespoonfuls butter, three tablespoonfuls cream and a little salt and pepper.

Have ready small tin pans lined with puff paste, into each of which put three or four oysters and some of the liquor, cover with paste and bake twenty minutes in a quick oven.

---

*For Open Patties*, cut the paste into round cakes; those intended for the bottom crust less than half an inch thick, for the upper crust one inch, from the latter cut a hole in the center, leaving a neat ring. Place this ring on the lower crust and another ring above this, that quite a cup may be formed. Lay the pieces cut out, in the oven with the "shells" and bake to a light brown. When done glaze with white of egg and return to the oven for three minutes. Fill the "shells" with the following: Add to half the liquor from a quart of oysters an equal quantity of milk and let it come to a boil. Put in all the oysters leaving out the uncooked liquor, heat to a boiling and stir in one tablespoonful butter and two tablespoonfuls of, corn starch, wet with a little milk and put in a little salt, boil four minutes stirring constantly until it thickens. Fill the "shell" with this, fitting on the top tightly. Mrs. C. P. Humphrey.

---

*Pickled Oysters.*—Take one hundred and fifty large oysters, look them over, and put in a large porcelain kettle with the liquor, put in a little salt when you put them on the fire as it helps to make them firm, let them remain until they boil up and appear plump, then take out the oysters and add to the liquor, one pint of vinegar, one tablespoonful of mace, one teaspoonful of cloves, and one of pepper grass and let it boil, let the oysters get cold and then turn over them the liquor, also cold. They are better the second day. The spices should not be ground.

Mrs. Humphrey.

*Oyster Croquettes.*—Heat to a scalding one-half pint sweet cream with a pinch of soda, thicken with one tablespoonful of butter rubbed smooth in four teaspoonfuls of corn starch, stirring constantly. When thick add one quart of oysters minced fine, with salt, pepper and lemon juice to taste, cooking not more than five minutes. When stiff and cold, mould with floured hands, into croquettes. Let them stand in a cool place for three or four hours then dip into egg and bread crumbs and fry in hot lard.

Mrs. Marvin.

*Escalloped Oysters.*—Cover the bottom of a well buttered pan with rolled crackers or bread crumbs, add a layer of oysters seasoned with salt, pepper and plenty of butter; then another layer of crumbs, then oysters till the pan is full, the last layer being crumbs, dotted with bits of butter. Pour over the whole the oyster liquid with milk added enough to moisten, cover and bake for half an hour.

Mrs. F. S. Newton.

*Friccassed Oysters.*—Drain one quart of oysters through a colander then set them into a spider in which four tablespoonfuls of butter have been browned. Stir into the oysters four tablespoonfuls of cream mixed smooth with one tablespoonful of flour. Before taking from the stove stir in the well beaten yolks of four eggs, being careful that it shall not boil after the eggs are added.

Mrs. J. G. Raymond.

*Oyster Fritters.*—Drain off the liquor, which boil and skim, then add to each cupful of liquor, one cupful of milk, two well beaten eggs, salt and pepper to taste, flour to make moderately stiff batter. Drop into hot lard from a large spoon taking an oyster in each spoonful of batter.

Mrs. A. J.

*Oyster Omelet.*—Beat six eggs very light, separately, season with pepper and salt, add two tablespoonfuls of cream with a good tablespoonful of butter. Drop into the omelet eight or ten large oysters chopped fine and fry. Fold over and send to the table at once.

Mrs. C. Johnston.

*Little Pigs in Blankets.*—Carefully wrap a large oyster in a thin slice of pork, using a toothpick to fasten, then broil.

Mrs. Adams.

*Fried Frogs.*—Parboil the hind quarters three or four minutes to which a teaspoonful of vinegar or lemon juice has been added, wipe dry, dip in bread crumbs then into egg, then into bread crumbs again, fry in smoking hot fat for one minute.

Mrs. W. C. Jacobs.

---

*Codfish a la Mode.*—Mix well together, one teacup codfish picked fine, two cups of mashed potato, one pint of milk, two well beaten eggs, one-half teacup butter, salt and pepper to taste, and bake twenty-five minutes. Mrs. W. J. Ellis.

---

*Broiled Oysters.*—Grease the griddle with a piece of salt pork. Drain the oysters carefully then lay them on the griddle, a bit of butter to each oyster, turn and serve immediately on buttered toast. Mrs. Adams.

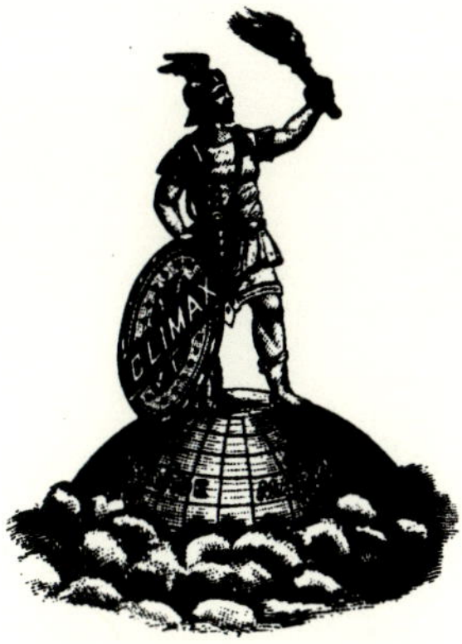


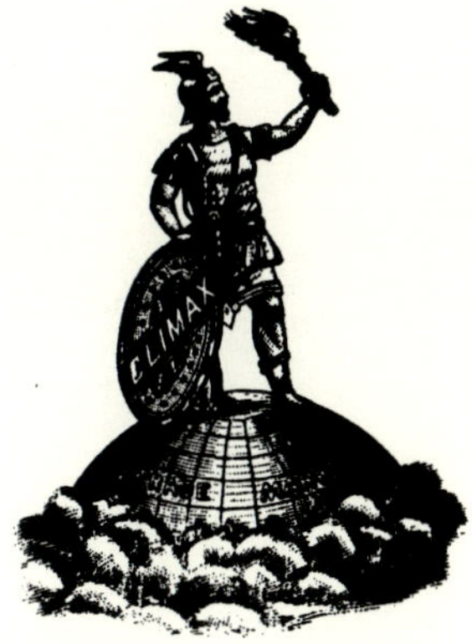


# TAPLIN, RICE & Co.

**AKRON, OHIO.**

—MANUFACTURE A GENERAL ASSORTMENT OF—

# STOVES

Especially designed for this market, among which is their celebrated line of

## CLIMAX COOKS AND HEATERS,

*The acknowledged Leaders of the Stove Market.*

**New Cooking Range and several other patterns nearly ready.**

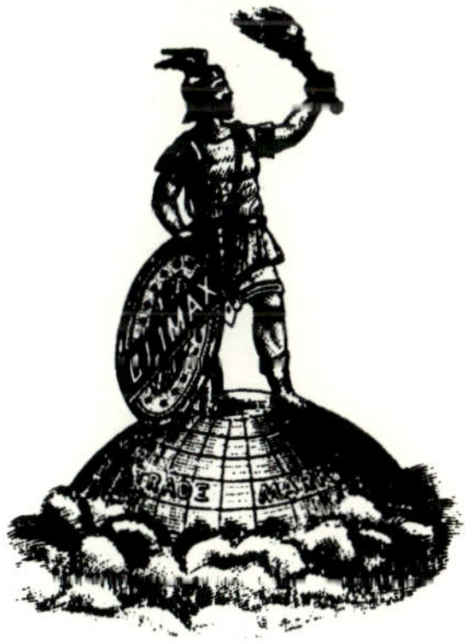


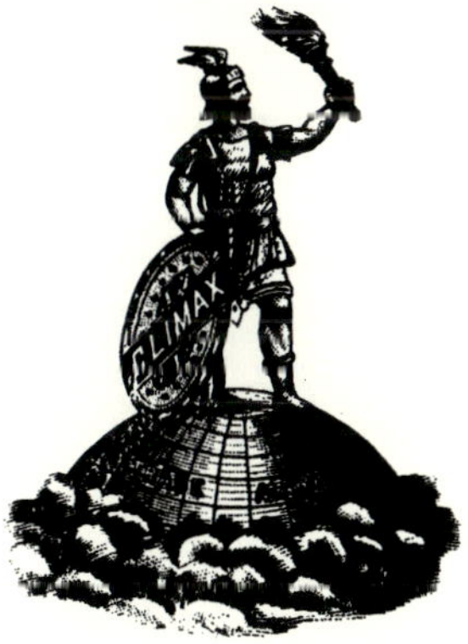

# MEATS.

" Venison's a Cæsar in the fiercest fray,
Turtle, an Alexander in its way ;
And then in quarrels of a slighter nature,
Mutton's a most successful mediator ;
So much superior is the stomach's smart
To all the vaunted horrors of the heart ;
E'en love, who often triumphs, is his grief,
Hath ceased to feed on sighs, to pant on beef."

*To Roast a Turkey.*—A turkey a year old is considered the best, see that it is well washed. salt and pepper it inside, put into a dripping pan, salt and pepper outside, sprinkle flour over it. Roast about three hours in a moderate oven, be sure and keep an even fire.

---

*Plain Stuffing for Turkey.*—Take stale bread, cut off all the crust, rub very fine and pour over it as much melted butter as will make it crumble in your hand, salt and pepper to your taste, add small quantity of onion and sage if agreeable.

---

*Turkey Dressing with Oysters.*—For a ten-pound turkey take two pints of bread crumbs, half a teacupful of butter, one teaspoonful of each sage, pepper and salt, mix thoroughly, rub the turkey well inside and out with salt and pepper, then fill with first a spoonful of crumbs, then a few well drained oysters using half a can for the turkey, strain the oyster liquor and use to baste the turkey, cook the giblets and chop fine for the gravy. A fowl of this size will require three hours cooking in a moderate oven.

---

*Baked Beefsteak.*—Take a tender round of beefsteak cut about an inch thick, make stuffing as for turkey and roll it up in the meat, bake until very tender.

---

*Breakfast Dish.*—Chop very fine either cold beef, mutton or veal. To one teacupful allow the same quantity of grated bread, to this quantity add one egg yolk and white well beaten together, salt, pepper and if liked a very small onion chopped fine, mix well together and flour your hands, make into balls and fry in hot lard.

---

*Stewed Tongue.* Boil a beef's tongue in a little water seasoned with salt and pepper. When nearly tender, remove it from the kettle and skin, saving the liquor to make the gravy. The following day cut the tongue in half, lengthwise, stick a clove in each half, put it into a kettle, with a gravy, made according to the receipt given elsewhere for brown gravy; add one very small onion, cover closely, and let it cook very slowly for an hour, or till it is tender. Place the cut sides on the platter and the roots of the tongue together, the tips pointing in the same direction. Pour the gravy, having removed the bits of onion, over the tongue. Garnish the edge of the platter with large slices cut from cucumber pickles. This dish is ornamental to the table, and generally well liked. Mrs. R. H. Wright.

---

*French Method of Making Gravy.*—Put a large tablespoonful of butter into a skillet and place over the fire, adding when it foams up two tablespoonfuls of flour. Stir and blend constantly, till it becomes a rich brown, but it must not burn. When the roast is cooked, take it from the dripping pan and place on a platter. With a spoon remove all grease from the dripping pan, then slowly pour the remaining liquor into the browned flour, stirring constantly, seasoning to taste. Mrs. R. H. Wright.

---

*Veal Cutlets.*—Remove all bits of skin, sinew and vein from uncooked veal; chop it very fine with a little parsley, salt and pepper. The mince should now be made into the shape of cutlets, which must be dipped first into bread crumbs, then into well-beaten egg, then into crumbs, covering nicely on both sides; fry in boiling lard or butter, and serve with spinach, sorrel, green peas, asparagus, or tomatoes. N. S.

---

*To Cook Veal Steak.*—Cut into pieces about half an inch square, removing all strings, fat and gristle. Put into a spider one tablespoonful butter and one of lard, let it get very hot, and turn in the meat, stirring constantly until browned. Do not let it stew but fry. Have ready one tablespoonful of flour in a sifter, sprinkle the meat with pepper and salt, sift the flour over and stir until brown, turn on one pint of milk, let come to a boil and serve. If the butter be not seething hot, the juices will stew out of the meat. Mrs. Latham.

---

*To Cook Veal Steak.*—Wipe the steaks dry, then dip them into rolled cracker, then into beaten egg, then into the cracker again; lay carefully into a spider in which a half teacupful of butter is very hot, when browned on on one side turn gently. When both sides are well browned, cover closely, having sprinkled salt, pepper and curry powder on the meat, and set where they will cook slowly twenty minutes. When well done, take the meat from the spider, stir in the butter a cup of milk in which has been stirred smooth a large spoonful of flour, or sifted crumbs, let it boil two minutes, and pour over the meat. Miss Angel.

*Pot Pie.*—Boil in plenty of water seven or eight lbs. of veal, with the bone, skimming it nicely. Take enough dough for a loaf of bread, work into it shortening as for biscuit, and let it rise. When light, roll out and let it rise again, pricking as biscuit. Season the broth highly, and drop in the biscuits, let it boil three-fourths of an hour, keeping closely covered.

When dishing pull apart carefully the biscuits, putting them on the top of the meat. Mrs. J. A. M.

---

*Croquettes.*—Boil together one cup each of bread crumbs and milk, adding salt and pepper to taste. When nearly cold, add one cup chopped beef, and mould into croquettes. Put in a cool place for an hour, then dip into beaten egg and bread crumbs and fry in hot lard. Mrs. Mabley.

---

*Veal Steak.*—Cut in pieces, dip in egg, then bread crumbs, and fry in hot lard. Season with salt, pepper, the juice and bit of the rind of a lemon, cooking very slow. Place on dish, putting bits of butter on the meat, thicken the gravy, and pour over the meat and serve.

---

*Yorkshire Pudding.*—Twenty minutes before the roast of beef is done, pour off the gravy and dip around the meat, but not touching it, two eggs beaten light, one pint sweet milk and flour to make a thin batter, return to the oven and cook twenty minutes. Serve with the meat. Mrs. J. P. Boyd.

---

*To Cook Ham or Corned Beef.*—Cover the meat with a paste of flour and water and bake slowly in oven five hours.

---

*Stuffing for Veal.*—Bread crumbs, egg sufficient to moisten, salt, pepper, lemon juice and a little of the peel, chopped parsley, and butter size of a small egg. Mrs. J. Boyd.

---

*Stewed Beef*—Put ribs of beef into a kettle, brown well both sides, then add water, salt, pepper, a little whole allspice and a small carrot. Stew three or four hours; when done thicken the gravy, and serve. Mrs. J. P. Boyd.

---

*Fried Calves' Liver.*—Cut the liver in thin slices, dip the slices into flour and fry slowly in hot butter, seasoning with salt, pepper and a little summer savory. When done add a little tomato catsup to the gravy. Mrs. J. Boyd.

---

*Spiced Veal.*—Three pounds veal, eight butter crackers, two eggs, a piece of butter size of an egg, one tablespoonful salt, one tablespoonful black pepper. Chop the veal fine. roll the crackers and mix well together and make into the form of a loaf or roll, put into a dripping pan and bake slowly two hours, basting with melted butter occasionally. Cut in thin slices and serve.

Mrs. Humphrey.

---

*To Fry Calves' Liver.*—Remove the skin from the liver, cut in strips an inch in thickness, lay them in milk over night or several hours. Take them from the milk, dip them in beaten egg and then in bread crumbs, in which a little salt has been mixed. Fry in hot butter, and serve with minced parsley.

---

*Sweet Breads.*—Soak them in salt water over night, in the morning boil them until tender in water and butter. Let the water boil down and the butter brown on them, then slice them, roll in eggs and cracker twice and fry in half butter and lard.

Mrs. Humphrey.

---

*Ham Sandwiches.*—Half teacup of vinegar, two eggs, one large tablespoonful of butter, two heaping tablespoonfuls white sugar, two even tablespoonfuls mustard, a little salt, boil this together and when partially cold pour it over half a ham chopped fine. Butter thin slices of bread, spread with the ham and fold them.

Mrs. Humphrey.

---

*Pot Pie.*—Stew in plenty of water seven or eight pounds of veal, or rabbit, (if the latter put a little vinegar into the water), skimming nicely. About half an hour before dinner, make a dough of one quart flour in which *four* full teaspoonfuls baking powder have been thoroughly sifted, a piece of butter size of walnut, salt, and cold water to make a stiff dough. Drop from the spoon into the stew, which *must be boiling* and *kept* so twenty minutes. The cover must not be removed till done. The biscuits will be as dry as if baked, if taken up at once. Miss Angel.

---

*Veal Loaf.*—Mix very thoroughly together, three and one-half pounds of veal, very finely minced, fat and lean, three well beaten eggs, one tablespoonful pepper, one and one half tablespoonful salt, one nutmeg, a cup of sifted rolled crackers, butter size of an egg, three tablespoonfuls cream, mold into a loaf and bake two hours. Mrs. R. H. Wright.

---

*Veal Loaf.*—Mince very fine, fat and lean together, three and one-half lbs., of veal and mix thoroughly with three well beaten eggs, crackers, rolled fine, one tablespoonful pepper.

---

*Yorkshire Pudding.*—About thirty minutes before roast beef is to be served, remove it from the pan, pour off the greater part of the drippings, and return it to oven. Have ready one and a half pints of milk into which has been stirred the beaten yolks of three eggs, a pinch of salt, and six tablespoonfuls of flour, adding last the beaten whites of eggs and pour into pan with meat. Cut into blocks and serve nicely piled on a small platter.

Miss A. J.

---

*Creamed Sweetbreads.*—Parboil as for broiling dropped into cold water, and wiped dry, cut into dice, heated in seasoned white sauce, and serve on toasted bread. Miss A. J.

---

*Frizzle Beef.*—Shave off thin slices of dried beef, put into a spider and pour on a little warm water, stir up and turn off the water, add a piece of butter the size of an egg to a pound of beef, put the whole over the fire, beat two eggs with three tablespoonfuls of milk, dredge the beef with a little flour, pour over it the eggs and milk, let it come to a boil and serve. Mrs. Humphrey.

---

*Veal Loaf.*—Mix three pounds finely chopped veal, with butter size of an egg, three well-beaten eggs, three tablespoonfuls cream, thoroughly together, then add four square soda crackers, powdered, one tablespoonful pepper, one tablespoonful salt, same quantity of sage. Bake two and a half hours, basting with butter. Mrs. W. J. Ellis.

---

*Hash.*—Mix two-thirds cold potato, chopped very fine, and one-third meat, season with salt, pepper and finely minced onion; place in pan and dredge with a little flour, and pour in on the side enough water to come up even with the hash. Place it in the oven, but do not stir. When the flour has formed a crust, take from the oven, add a lump of butter and stir it through several times. Mrs. W. J. E.

---

*Escalloped Chicken.*—Boil two large chickens with a piece of pork, cut into small pieces and season with salt, pepper and butter. Chop fine one pint of oysters, mix with chicken and prepare the same as escalloped oysters. Mrs. F. S. N.

---

*Chicken Croquettes.*—Chop four chickens, (or any meat, except beef,) as fine as possible, add one-fourth as much bread crumbs as there is chopped meat, one egg to each cup full of meat and crumbs. If egg is not desireable, cream or drawn butter may be used instead. Season to taste with salt, pepper, chopped parsley, or celery, make into small cakes, keeping them as soft as possible, insert in one end of each cake a small piece of macaroni, and fry in hot butter. Mrs. F. S. Newton.

---

*Veal Croquettes.*—One-half pound veal or chicken, chopped very fine, fry one-fourth grated onion in one tablespoonful butter, stir the onion until yellow, add one tablespoonful of flour, stir a few minutes longer, then add a coffeecupful of broth in which the veal has been cooked, (more, if needed,) stir in the chopped veal, and salt to taste. Cook ten minutes, stiring all the time, put in a little grated nutmeg and cayenne pepper, stir in yolks of two eggs, give it one hard boil, and put in dish to cook. When cold, form into balls and dip in cracker dust and white or yolk of an egg; great care must be taken to have the lard boiling hot, and plenty of it; dip the balls in carefully, three or four at a time. Cook until a light brown. Mrs. C. E. Perkins.

---

*Veal or Chicken Croquettes.*—One pint finely minced veal or chicken, well seasoned with salt and pepper, use this with a dressing, made as follows: two tablespoonfuls of butter brought to a boiling point, in which stir two tablespoonfuls of flour, then a half pint of milk, stirring till it is a perfectly smooth paste. Remove from fire, add one well beaten egg, two teaspoonfuls lemon juice, one teaspoonful minced parsley, one saltspoonful celery salt, one half saltspoonful salt, a little white pepper and a few drops onion juice. After thoroughly mixing meat and dressing, spread on a platter to cool and harden, after which make into croquettes. Roll first in sifted bread crumbs or rolled cracker, then in yolk of egg, to which is added one tablespoonful of water, again in crumbs, then fry in deep fat, as for doughnuts, one minute. Mrs. W. C. Jacobs.

---

*Chicken Pie.*—Stew the fowls until tender, season to taste and thicken the gravy. Line the sides of the baking pan with a paste made by rubbing into a scant quart of flour, into which three teaspoonfuls of baking powder have been sifted, two-thirds of a cup of shortening, mixed soft with cold water; put in the chicken, cover with the paste rolled moderately thick, *being careful to make openings in the cover.* Mrs. Mary Baker.

---

*Ham Balls.*—Cold boiled ham chopped fine, as many well-beaten eggs as there are persons, flour to beat together and make into balls, which are to be fried in hot butter.

Mrs. P. W. Leavitt.

---

*Chicken Cheese.*—Boil an old chicken thoroughly in sufficient water to cover it; chop fine, and having boiled down the water to a cupful, put in the chopped chicken, cook a few minutes, season with salt and pepper, put into a mold and set on the ice to cool. Mrs. N. Monsarrat.

E. R. HULL. S. E GRAVES. J. C. McWATTERS.

# E. R. HULL & CO.

**OHIO'S GREATEST CLOTHIERS,**

Have opened a Branch Store

→ AT ←

## 163 and 165 South Howard Street,

AKRON, O.

---

WE CARRY THE LARGEST ASSORTMENT OF

## Men's, Youth's and Children's Clothing

**HATS, CAPS AND**

**FURNISHING GOODS.**

---

**We Sell at the same LOW PRICES that has made our Main Store so popular in Northern Ohio.**

YOU are invited to give us a call. You will not be importuned to buy unless you wish to. We take pleasure in showing our stock to any and all callers.

## E. R. HULL & CO.,

**163-165 South Howard Street, - - AKRON, OHIO.**

**G. H. MACEY, Manager.**

STORES.—Cleveland, Youngstown, Newburgh and Akron.

# SALADS.

*Sydney Smith's Recipe for Salad Dressing.*—

"Two boiled potatoes strained through a kitchen sieve,
Softness and smoothness to the salad give;
Of mordant mustard take a single spoon;
Distrust the condiment that bites too soon;
Yet deem it not, thou man of taste, a fault,
To add a double quantity of salt.
Four times the spoon with oil of Lucca crown,
And twice with vinegar procured from town,
True taste requires it, and your poet begs
The pounded yellow of two well boiled eggs.
Let onion's atoms lurk within the bowl,
And scarce suspected stimulate the whole;
And, lastly, in the flavored compound toss
A magic spoonful of anchovy sauce.
Oh, great and glorious! Oh, herbaceous meat!
'Twould tempt the dying anchorite to eat.
Back to the world he'd turn his weary soul
And plunge his fingers in the salad bowl."

*Salmon Salad.*—Cover a platter with crisp lettuce, over which spread a can of salmon. Pour over this a dressing of one cup of sour cream or milk, two tablespoonfuls mustard, salt and pepper, cooked slowly with one and a half cups vinegar, two eggs well beaten, stirred in while cooking, adding butter size of a walnut. When cool pour over the salmon, covering the top with slices of lemon Mrs. Thomas Robinson.

---

*Salad Dressing.*—Stir into three tablespoonfuls of olive oil, a spoonful of salt. Beat the yolks of two eggs very light, then stir in six tablespoonfuls of vinegar, teaspoonful of sugar, and pepper to taste, oil and salt. Cook until thick. Just before sending to the table add half a cup of thick or whipped cream.

Mrs. D. L. King.

---

*Salad Dressing.*—One tablespoonful of flour, one half tablespoonful of French mustard, three tablespoonfuls of cream, six tablespoonfuls of vinegar, two eggs, well beaten, butter size of an egg, salt and pepper. Beat well together and cook till quite thick. Prepare as follows; mix flour and cream together, mustard and vinegar, beat eggs light and add melted butter, then cream and flour, last add vinegar and mustard. Stir constantly. Miss King.

---

*Sweetbread Salad.*—Boil the sweetbreads twenty minutes, when cold, split them and fry a nice brown in butter. Break into small pieces, add lettuce, and dressing made by pouring half bottle of olive oil in a thread sized stream, into yolks of two eggs, two tablespoonfuls vinegar, two teaspoonfuls mixed mustard, stirring constantly. Mrs. D. L. King.

*Oyster Salad.*—One quart oysters, one small onion, celery, one raw egg, yolks of two hard boiled eggs, two tablespoonfuls olive oil, one teaspoonful sugar, one half spoonful each of pepper, salt and made mustard, half a cupful vinegar. Whip the raw eggs light with butter and oil and add the hard eggs rubbed to a paste with the salt, pepper, and mustard and beat in the vinegar, a few drops at a time. Drain the oysters, cut them into small pieces also the celery. Put oysters and celery into a salad bowl, mix with half the dressing, pour the rest over it.

*Salmon Salad.*—Set a can of salmon in a kettle of boiling water, letting it boil twenty minutes, when take from the can, pouring off all the oil. Put in a deep dish, putting in a few cloves, sprinkle with salt and pepper, cover with cold vinegar letting stand all day. When ready to use, take from the vinegar, and place on a platter, cover with dressing made of yolks of two hard boiled eggs worked to a paste with a tablespoonful mustard, three of melted butter, a little salt and pepper, with the yolks of two eggs well beaten. Mix this thoroughly, adding slices of peeled lemon. Mrs. Neri Newcomb.

*Salad Dressing, (Without Oil.)*—Scald together one half cup vinegar, one cup butter and add four eggs well beaten, one half pint milk or cream, one tablespoonful mixed mustard, a little salt and stir until thick. Mrs. J. A. Mason.

*Pickled Cabbage.*—To each head of cabbage, slawed fine, add one cup of sugar, one tablespoonful ground mustard, three green peppers, chopped fine, one tablespoonful salt, celery to taste or five cents worth of celery salt, and cover with vinegar.

Sarah Buckingham.

*Potato Salad.*—Slice very thin, cold boiled or steamed potatoes, season well with salt and white pepper. To every three potatoes use one hard boiled egg and one cucumber. Slice in the dish the potatoes, eggs and cucumber in alternate layers, covering each with dressing, being very careful not to stir as this makes the salad look "mussy," nor be stingy with the dressing, using it with a lavish hand on top.

*Dressing.*—Well beaten yolks of five eggs in five tablespoonfuls of boiling vinegar, cooking bowl set in water, stirring constantly until thick when remove from the fire and add four ounces butter, stirring till cool and smooth, one teaspoonful of French mustard, one teaspoonful onion juice or finely minced onion, one teaspoonful minced parsley. When ready to use on the salad, thin with cream, until it will just pour. Mrs. W. C. Jacobs.

---

*Salmon Salad.*—Fill a good sized platter with the inside leaves of a head of lettuce, and spread over this the salmon picked apart with a fork.

The dressing is made of one cup of sour cream, two tablespoonfuls of sugar, one tablespoonful of mustard, salt and pepper to taste—cayenne is better than black—one half cup of vinegar, three eggs well beaten, and stirred into the cream, then add sugar, salt, mustard and pepper. Put on the stove and cook as for cabbage, while hot add butter size of a large walnut, when cold pour over the salmon. Mrs. G. T. Perkins.

---

*Governor's Sauce.*—Chop fine together one peck of green tomatoes, eight green peppers and four onions, to this add one cup of salt, and let it stand over night. In the morning drain off the juice, add one cup of sugar, one-fourth pound yellow mustard seed, one tablespoonful each of cloves and cinnamon, cover with vinegar and cook gently for two hours. When cool add one cup grated horseradish. Mrs. G. Johnston.

---

*Prepared Mustard.*—Mix smooth with hot water three teaspoonfuls of ground mustard, one-half teaspoonful sugar, one teaspoonful flour, a little salt, add a little vinegar.

---

*Chili Sauce.*—Eighteen ripe tomatoes, pared, three green peppers, one large onion, one cup sugar, two and one-half cups vinegar, two teaspoonfuls salt, one of cinnamon, one of cloves. Cook the tomatoes tender, chop the onion and peppers very fine, mix all, and cook a few minutes.

---

*Oyster Sauce.*—Put the oysters into a saucepan and heat slowly in the strained liquor, but not boil. After they have simmered a few minutes, take out the oysters, stir into the liquor a quarter of a pound of butter, beaten smooth with a tablespoonful of flour, and as it boils add a breakfast cup of cream, stirring constantly. Add the oysters and remove to the back of the stove till wanted. Serve with fowl, or use for filling oyster patties.

---

*Potted Ham.*—Cut the remnants of boiled ham into small pieces, and pound to a paste in a mortar, softening with a little melted butter. Add cayenne pepper to taste, and put into small bowls or jars, pressing closely and smooth. Pour over a little melted butter, cover closely, and set away. This will keep for weeks. Mrs. J. A. Mason.

*Pickled Eggs.*—Boil the eggs very hard; when cool, cut in halves, lengthwise. Sprinkle them plentifully with vinegar to which has been added a little melted butter, pepper and salt.

Mrs. R. R. Smith.

---

*Devilled Eggs.*—Boil eggs thirty minutes, shell them, cut lengthwise, remove yolks. Scald together butter and small quantity of vinegar, to which add yolks with mustard, salt and pepper mixed. Put back into whites. Good for lunch.

Mrs. P. R. Smith.

---

*Devilled Eggs.*—Boil six eggs ten minutes, put into cold water, peel, cut in halves, slicing a little off one end, so that the egg will stand up. Remove the yolks; rub them to a smooth paste with a little melted butter, cayenne pepper, mustard and vinegar, with which fill the hollows in the whites, and serve in bed of white cabbage, sliced, or use as granish for meats.

Mrs. Howard.

---

*Cold Catsup.*—One-half peck ripe tomatoes, chopped, drained, one pint chopped celery, one small onion, one-half ounce white mustard seed, three red peppers, chopped, two teaspoonfuls cinnamon, same quantity each of cloves and pepper corns, one-half cup salt. Stir all together with vinegar to cover, and bottle.

Mrs. Keniston.

---

*Mint Sauce.*—Chop three tablespoonfuls mint, add a heaping tablespoonful sugar, and one-half coffee cup of vinegar. Stir while heating and serve when cold with roast lamb.

Mrs. J. A. M.

---

*Dressing for Sandwiches.*—Beat together halt a pound of butter, three tablespoonfuls mixed mustard, same of oil, a little white or red pepper, salt, the yolk of one egg, and set on ice, chop very fine ham and tongue, (a little chicken is an improvement.) Cut the bread very thin, spread on it first the dressing then the meat. Cover with a slice of bread, pressed down closely. Trim the edges, making the sandwiches as nearly one size as possible.

Mrs. F. S. Newton.

---

*Cheese Scollop.*—Soak one cup bread crumbs in fresh milk, into this beat three eggs, add one tablespoonful butter, and one-half ponnd grated cheese. Strew over the top sifted bread crumbs, and bake in the oven a delicate brown.

Mrs. P. R. Smith.

---

*Potato Salad.*—Six large, cold boiled potatoes, cut into small pieces, onion to taste, (celery can be substituted,) two hard boiled eggs chopped fine with onion. Pour over this two large spoonfuls vinegar, one-half cup butter, scalded together; two eggs well beaten, one small cup of cream or milk, one teaspoonful mixed mustard, salt and pepper, stirred to the consistency of thick cream.

Mrs. J. A. Mason.

---

*Welsh Rarebit.*—Melt together in a saucepan, four tablespoonfuls sherry, (the California wine will answer very well,) and a piece of butter size of a butternut, then add a coffeecupful of grated cheese, which should be rich and of medium age, four tablespoonfuls of milk and a little cayenne pepper—a teaspoonful grated horseradish is an improvement—and boil together a few minntes. Have ready some slices of bread with the crust removed, toasted and buttered on one side; lay on each piece a thin slice of mild, rich cheese; set in the oven till it melts; place on hot dish, pour over it the above mixture, and serve immediately.

H. C. Gaylord, Cleveland.

---

*Escalloped Eggs.*—Put into a buttered baking dish a layer ot bread crumbs, moistened with milk or meat broth. Add to half a teacup of drawn butter (for five eggs) a well beaten egg; into this dip slices of hard boiled eggs, of which make a layer on the bread crumbs, sprinkling with minced ham, veal or chicken; then another layer of crumbs, covered with eggs, meat, etc., having crumbs as a cover. Bake twenty minutes in a moderate oven.

Miss Francis.

---

*Eggs Au Plat.*—Into a large, well buttered pie plate pour a cup of rich cream, and break into this ten eggs, being careful to keep them whole. Sprinkle a little salt, pepper and bits of butter over the top; set in oven long enough to brown over the top, but do not cook too long, as they will continue to harden on the hot plate after being removed from the oven. The eggs should be solid enough to be eaten with a fork, but no harder. Serve in the dish in which they are baked. Mrs. R. H. Wright.

# P. L. MILES & CO.

Wholesale and Retail Dealers in

# DIAMONDS

AND OTHER PRECIOUS STONES.

—ALSO—

## Watches, Clocks,
## Jewelry and
## Silver Ware.

Manufacturers of all kinds of GOLD AND SILVER JEWELRY and PRESENTATION BADGES.

## DIAMOND SETTING

A SPECIALTY.

When in the city give us a call and we will be pleased to show our large assortment at

**9 Euclid Avenue, CLEVELAND, OHIO.**

## ANNOUNCEMENT.

# L. A. BARMORE,

**154 & 156 S. Main St., Akron, O.,**

Is ready with and invites inspection of the CHOICEST LINE of chaste designs in

# Fine and Medium Furniture

IN THIS MARKET.

See the beautiful Antique Bedroom Suits, Sideboards, Book-cases, Chiffeniers, Hall Stands, Phœnix Folding Beds,

## PARLOR SUITS

In all woods and coverings, DINING ROOM, LIBRARY AND OFFICE FURNITURE in all the popular woods.

TELEPHONE NO. 262. **L. A. BARMORE.**

---

# THE WHITE IS KING!

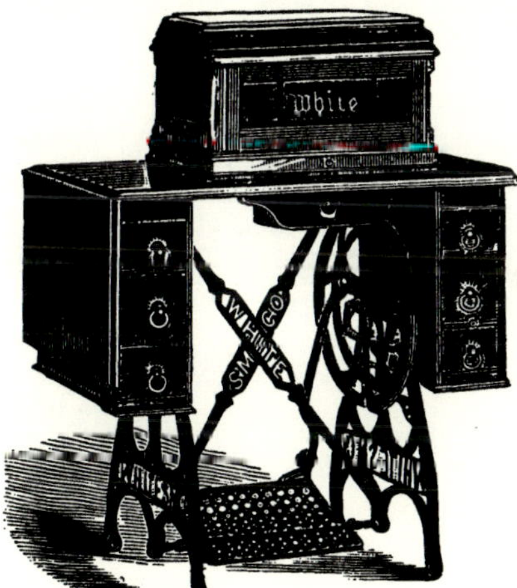


PERFECT, POWERFUL,

POPULAR, SIMPLE,

SILENT, SURE.

## 600,000

## White Sewing Machines

**NOW IN USE.**

We make the WHITE upon principles of

## DURABILITY,

And Warrant it for Five Years.

For Circulars and Particulars, address

**WHITE SEWING MACHINE CO., Cleveland, Ohio.**

## USE

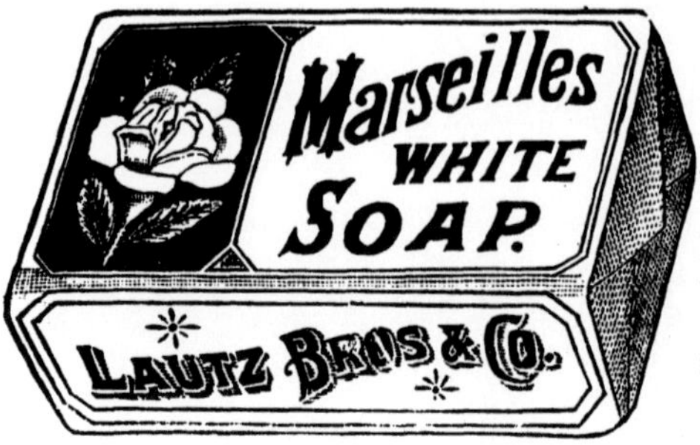


**MARSEILLES WHITE SOAP**
is unexcelled for
**Washing Flannels.**
It will not "full up" as when washed with ordinary Soap, and will remain
SOFT AND BEAUTIFUL.

**SAVE YOUR MARSEILLES SOAP WRAPPERS!**

Mail us 15 Colored Marseilles Soap Wrappers and we will send you a handsome set of PICTURE CARDS.

**LAUTZ BROS. & CO., Buffalo, N. Y.**

---

## USE

**—BEST—**
**BAR SOAP**
**MADE.**

Cut Full Pound.

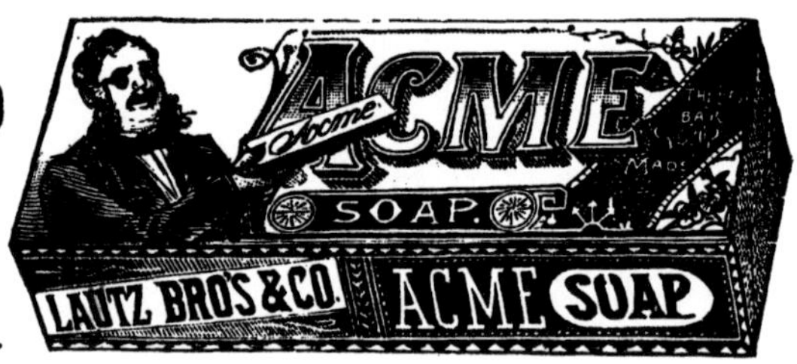


**SAVE YOUR ACME WRAPPERS!**

Mail us 15 Colored Acme Wrappers and we will send you a handsome set of PICTURE CARDS.

**LAUTZ BROS. & CO., Buffalo, N. Y.**

# VEGETABLES.

**No life worth naming ever comes to good,
If always nourished on the self-same food.**

*Boston Baked Beans.*—Use the smallest white bean; soak over night. In the morning add fresh cold water, let parboil one hour, slowly. Put in bean pot, allowing to one quart beans one pound salt pork, (fat,) three tablespoonfuls molasses. Fill bean pot with boiling water, replenishing all day as it boils out, until one and one-half hour before serving. Bake in moderate oven. Beans should be a light brown when done. The proper bean pot is smaller at the top than the bottom; can be found at all potteries. Bake twelve or fourteen hours. Mrs. J. A. Mason.

---

*Macaroni and Cheese.*—Wash the macaroni, and put into boiling milk and water for fifteen minutes; drain into a colander, cut into pieces an inch long, and put a layer into a large pudding dish, then a layer of grated cheese, with a sprinkle of dry mustard, or curry, salt and butter, then a layer of macaroni, then the cheese, etc., thus filling the dish, the cheese being the top layer, and bake a good half hour in a quick oven. Mrs. Howard.

**"And e'en if the moon be not made of green cheese,
There are some good things that are, if you please."**

---

*Schmier-Kaese.*—Take thick milk, heat it just a little, then put in a bag and hang up to let all the whey drain off, then put it in a crock and stir it until fine. To a gallon of schmier-kaese add one quart of cream; salt to taste. N. B.

---

*Macaroni.*—Break into pieces an inch long the best Italian macaroni; when boiled soft, lay in a dish with alternate layers of grated cheese, bits of butter, pepper and salt, with grated cheese on the top. Pour over it a cup of milk and bake in a moderate oven till well browned. Mrs. J. A. Mason.

---

*Riced Potato.*—Heat a flat dish and the colander. With a spoon rub mashed potato through the colander, onto the hot dish, being careful that the colander does not touch the potato on the dish. It is best to put in but a few spoonfuls at once. When all has been pressed through, place the dish in the hot oven for five minutes.

In cooking turnips, beets, and the like, a little sugar is an improvement.

*Macaroni.*—Stew in salted water till soft one-half pound broken macaroni. When done, drain off the water, add a cup of cream or milk, a tablespoonful bread crumbs, made to a paste with two tablespoonfuls butter, teaspoonful curry, tablespoonful grated cheese, stew five minutes, set in the oven to brown.

Miss Angel.

---

*Cream Potatoes.*—Boil the potatoes in the skin. When cold, peel, chop fine; into a baking dish put a layer of potatoes, with salt, pepper and butter, then a layer of potatoes, repeating till the dish is full. Nearly cover them with sweet, rich cream and bake.

Mrs. C. E. Perkins.

---

*Potatoes Baked with Roast Beef.*—Pare the potatoes, cut in halves, lay around the meat in the dripping pan; about half an hour before serving sprinkle with salt and pepper and bake. Serve on the same platter as the meat, being placed around the edge.

---

*Boiled Potatoes.*—Twelve medium sized potatoes, one tablespoonful of salt, and boiling water to cover. Boil fifteen minutes, then add salt, and boil fifteen minutes longer. Pour off every drop of water. Take the cover from the saucepan and shake the potatoes in a current of air. Place the pan again on the stove and cover with a clean, coarse towel till serving.

---

*Escalloped Potatoes.*—Cover the bottom of a baking dish with a layer of cream sauce, then a layer of cold boiled potatoes sliced *very thin*, sprinkled with chopped parsley and moistened with sauce, continuing this till all the material is used, the last layer being the sauce. Cover with sifted crumbs, putting bits of butter on the top, and bake twenty minutes. One pint of sauce, one tablespoonful chopped parsley, half a cup of bread crumbs, salt and pepper to taste.

---

*Rice Cakes.*—One pint sweet milk, one pint cold boiled rice, a little melted butter, three well beaten eggs, a pinch of salt. Bake in iron gem pans thirty minutes. Mrs. C. E. Perkins.

---

*Corn Oysters.*—Beat well together one quart of grated corn, three yolks of eggs and three or four grated crackers, season with salt and pepper and beat in, just before frying in hot lard, the whites, whipped stiff. Fry a light brown. Mrs. W. J. Ellis.

---

*A Cheese Relish.*—Four ounces of flour, four ounces of cheese, and three ounces of butter; knead together with salt and pepper and a dash of cayenne pepper, roll thin, cut in strips, and bake a delicate brown. Mrs. E. O. Stanley.

*Green Corn Pudding.*—One quart milk, six eggs, two tablespoonfuls melted butter, one tablespoonful white sugar, one can, or one dozen ears green corn. Beat the corn and yolks of eggs together, add milk and butter gradually, beating hard all the while, then sugar. a little salt, and lastly the whites beaten stiff. Bake slowly an hour, at first covered, then remove the cloth and brown.

Miss Carpenter.

---

*Corn Oysters.*—One pint grated sweet corn, one small teacup of flour, two eggs, one tablespoonful butter, salt and pepper. Drop from spoon into hot butter and fry brown. Mrs. Latham.

---

*Stewed Tomatoes.*—Stew as usual, when quite off the boil, stir in quickly three well beaten eggs. J. A. M.

---

*Potato Rolls.*—Boil and mash fine four large potatoes, adding a tablespoonful of butter and salt to taste, half a pint milk, half a teacup of yeast, with flour sufficient to make a dough; knead the dough, set it to rise when light, mold into little rolls, place on buttered tins to rise again, then bake. Miss Carpenter.

---

*Cooked Green Peppers.*—Wash the peppers thoroughly and cut out the seeds, fill with cold meat chopped fine, and bread crumbs, seasoned with salt, butter and pepper. Rub the ouside of each pepper with lard and bake half an hour.

Mrs. Fannie C. Wager.

---

*Stuffed Eggs.*—Boil hard one dozen eggs; when cold, cut into two parts. Mash the yolks thoroughly, adding pepper and salt to taste, two tablespoonfuls of salad oil, one dessert spoonful of tarragon vinegar, and a pinch of cayenne pepper, and replace in the cavities. Mrs. Fred. Ely, Cleveland.

---

*Rice Croquettes.*—One teacup of rice to one pint of milk, and one pint of water. Let cook in a crock until stiff. Mix with it, when cold, one egg. a spoonful melted butter, season with pepper and salt. Roll in balls with a little flour, and fry in hot lard, send to table hot. Mrs. C. H. Brown.

---

*Dressing for Sandwiches.*—One half pound nice butter, three tablespoonfuls of mixed mustard, three spoonfuls salad oil, the yolk of one hard boiled egg, rubbed to a smooth paste, with a little salt and pepper, then set on the ice to cool. Chop very fine any meat but beef, cut the bread very thin, spread it with dressing, then with meat, cover with bread, press closely, trim the edges, making the sandwiches one size. Mrs. G. T. Perkins.

2698.

# First National Bank.

T. W. CORNELL, President. W. McFARLIN, Cashier.

EDWARD OVIATT, Vice President. J. B. WRIGHT, Ass't Cash'r.

---

O. C. BARBER, President. T. W. CORNELL, Vice President. M. McFARLIN, Secretary and Treasurer.

# Portage Straw Board Co.

**WORKS:**
**NEW PORTAGE, OHIO.**

**OFFICE:**
**AKRON, OHIO.**

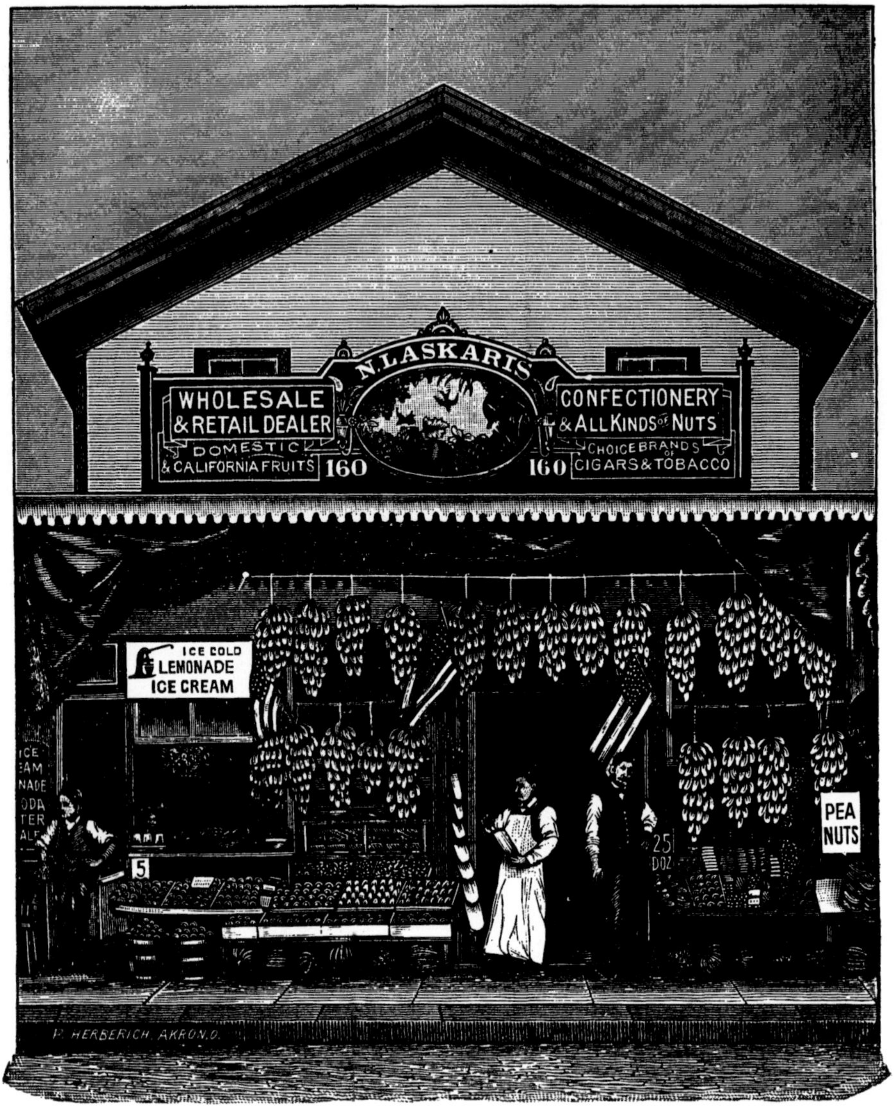


**Tropical Fruits, Nuts, Candies, &c., furnished for Parties and Weddings at all times, at Reasonable Prices.**

**L. LASKARIS,**

**TELEPHONE NO. 289.** **160 S. Howard St., AKRON, O.**

# DESSERTS.

" We buy ashes for bread;
We buy diluted wine;
Give me of the true, -
Whose ample leaves and tendrils curled
Among the silver hills of Heaven,
Draw everlasting dew.
Wine of wine,
Blood of the world,
Form of Forms, and mold of statures,
That I intoxicated,
And by the draught assimilated,
May float at pleasure through all natures,
The bird language rightly spell,
And that which roses say so well."—R. W. EMERSON.

*Chinese Method of Cooking Rice.*—Into a large milk pan of boiling water, slightly salted, scatter a cup of rice, (unwashed of course.) The pan must be sufficiently large to allow each grain to "crawl." Let it boil about twenty minutes, then turn into a sieve, that all the water may drain off, and serve. Chopsticks and bowls usually accompany this celestial dish, but it may be eaten with spoons if preferred. Mrs. R. H. Wright.

---

*Hard Sauce for Puddings.*—Beat well together one cup butter and three cups of sugar, adding any flavoring desired, and smooth into shape with a knife dipped into cold water.

---

*Banana Pudding.*—Cut stale sponge cake in slices, and place in a glass dish with alternate layers of sliced bananas, and pour over all a custard, made of yolks of eggs, milk and sugar, flavored with vanilla, covering the whole with the stiff beaten whites.

Mrs. J. H. Collins.

---

*Princess Pudding.*—Pour over alternate layers of thin bread and butter and any kind of canned fruit, (peaches are best,) a custard made of eggs and milk, proportioned to the size of the pudding pan, bake and eat with a sauce of butter and sugar beaten to a cream. Mrs. Carpenter.

---

*Whortleberry Pudding.*—One cup sugar, one half cup butter, two cups flour, one half cup milk, two eggs, one teaspoonful baking powder, one cup berries. Bake in small cake tins. Sauce:—Two cups sugar, one cup butter beaten to cream, one cup boiling water, whites three eggs. Flavor to taste, but sherry wine is best. Mrs. W. B. Raymond.

*Royal Diplomatic Pudding.*—Soak half a box of gelatine in half a cup of cold water two hours, then add two thirds of a pint of boiling water, the juice of a lemon, a cupful of sugar, and half a pint of sherry wine; stir thoroughly and strain. Have two molds, one holding two quarts, the other one quart. Put a layer of the jelly over the bottom of the large mold and place it on the ice. When hard garnish with candied cherries cut in halves, and pouring a few spoonfuls of liquid jelly (not hot,) to hold them, then pour in enough to cover them. Set again on the ice. When the jelly is perfectly hard, set the small mold in the center of the large one, filling the space between with jelly. Fill the small mold with ice, and set both in a basin of ice water. When the jelly is again hard, remove the ice from the small mold which fill with warm water and lift out carefully. Fill the vacant space with a custard made by the following recipe; soak half a box of gelatine in half a cup of cold water, then added to a scant cupful boiling milk, with the well beaten yolks of five eggs and half a cupful sugar, creamed with eggs, strain and add two tablespoonfuls wine, and one teaspoonful vanilla. When the custard begins to thicken add half a pint of cream, whipped to a froth. Pour this custard into the space mentioned and let it stand till it hardens. Turn the pudding out of the mold and serve with soft custard poured round it. Mrs. E. Steinbacher.

---

*Biron.*—Beat to a stiff froth the whites of four eggs and four tablespoonfuls of sugar, flavor with two thirds teaspoonful vanilla; pour over one third of a box of gelatine, dissolved in warm water, sufficient to cover it, beat till cold, put into a mold and set on the ice. Serve with cream. Miss Frank. R.

---

*Lemon Pudding.*—One quart of milk, two cups of bread crumbs, four eggs, one half cup of butter, one cup white sugar, two lemons, the rind of one grated. Soak the bread crumbs in the milk, and the beaten yolks and butter and sugar stirred to a cream, also the lemon. Bake until firm, then cover with a smering of the whites whipped to a stiff froth, with three tablespoonfuls powdered sugar, with a little lemon juice. Brown slightly. Orange pudding can be made the same way. Mrs. King.

---

*Steamed Pudding.*—Beat thoroughly together three eggs, tablespoonful of melted butter, salt, one cup sugar, one of sweet milk, three of flour, two tablespoonfuls baking powder, put into a buttered dish and steam two hours. Serve with wine sauce.

Miss Angel.

---

*Plain Cerealine Flake Pudding.*—Two cupfuls of scalded "Cerealine," cold, three eggs, two tablespoonfuls of sugar, half cupful of milk, half teaspoonful of salt, one tablespoonful of butter. Add the milk and butter to the "Cerealine" and rub it smooth; add the salt, sugar and nutmeg to suit the taste; beat the eggs to a light froth and stir into the mixture; put it into a well-buttered pudding dish and bake one-half hour, and serve hot with sweetened cream.

---

*Gelatine Pudding.*—Make a boiled custard with the yolks of four eggs, a pint of milk, and sugar to taste. Soak a third of a box of gelatine a few minutes in a little cold water, then dissolve it with three fourths of a cupful of boiling water. When the custard is cool, add the dissolved gelatine and beaten whites of the eggs and put into a mold. Serve with whipped cream.

Mrs. King.

---

*Pastry Cream.*—Two cupfuls of "Cerealine," two cupfuls of sugar, one tablespoonful of butter, one and a half pints of milk, two teaspoonfuls of vanilla, yolks of 5 eggs. Bring the milk to a boil with the sugar, and add the "Cerealine," as soon as it reboils take it from the fire, beat in the yolks, return to the fire two minutes to set the eggs; add the extract and butter, and use when cold.

---

*Puff Paste.*—One cupful of "Cerealine." two cupfuls of butter, one teaspoonful baking powder, one large cupful of ice-water, three cupfuls sifted flour, yolk of one egg, a little salt. Sift the flour with the baking powder, place it on a pastry-slab or mouldingboard then add the "Cerealine" and mix thoroughly, form the whole into a ring, place the egg-yolk and salt in the center. Add a little ice-water, and from the inside of the ring gradually take flour, adding ice-water every time until you have a smooth, firm paste, very tenacious and lithe. Place it on the ice for fifteen or twenty minutes, then roll out to the size of a dinner plate. Work the salt and butter milk out of the butter, and cut the butter in small pieces and place on the dough. Work the edges of the dough over the butter, carefully covering it. Turn it upside down, and roll out very thin; turn it back again and fold into a three square. Repeat the rolling and folding three times. Between each turn or operation of folding and rolling, put the dough on a thin tin, and place the tin on ice. As soon as it chills it will roll easily.

---

*Sauce for Sponge Pudding.*—Beat to a cream two cups of pulverized sugar and one-third of a cup of butter, then add one cup sweet cream, one nutmeg, one pint sherry wine; stir well and heat slowly in a pan set in hot water, but do not allow it to boil.

Mrs. Fred Ely, Cleveland.

---

*Small Almond Pudding.*—One-half pound sweet almonds, six bitter almonds, one-fourth pound sugar, two tablespoonfuls sifted sugar, two tablespoonfuls cream, one tablespoonful brandy. Blanch and beat the almonds to a paste with a spoonful of water; warm the butter and mix the almonds with this, and add the other ingredients, leaving out the whites of two eggs, mixing thoroughly. Butter some cups, half fill them and bake from twenty to thirty minutes. Turn them out and serve with sweet sauce.

Mrs. Alden.

---

*Sponge Pudding.*—One-fourth pound flour, one-fourth pound pulverized sugar, one-fourth pound butter, one quart milk, and sixteen eggs. Put the milk in a pail and set into a kettle of boiling water; mix the flour with cold milk reserved from the above, and stir into the milk when scalding hot, stirring briskly until it thickens, then add butter and sugar, not beaten, then the well beaten yolks of the eggs, lastly the whites, whipped to a stiff broth. Bake in a buttered pan about half an hour, setting the pan into a dish of water. Mrs. Fred Ely, Cleveland.

---

*English Plum Pudding.*—One pound each of currants, suet and sugar, two pounds raisins, one-half pound each of flour and bread crumbs, one-fourth of a candied orange and lemon peel, one teaspoonful of allspice, one nutmeg, one teaspoonful cinnamon, half a teaspoonful cloves, small teaspoonful salt, eight eggs, one-half pint sweet milk. Steam six hours. Mrs. Boyd.

---

*Fig Pudding.*—One-half pound figs, cut fine, six ounces each of bread crumbs, suet and sugar, three eggs, two teaspoonfuls cinnamon. Boil or steam two hours.

---

*Sauce.*—Beat well together two cups sugar, butter size of an egg, yolks of two eggs, put into a pan of water on the stove to melt, stirring all the time. Remove from the stove and stir in two or three tablespoonfuls of cream, add the whites well beaten, and set away to cool. Mrs. King.

---

*Puff Pudding.*—One coffeecup of flour, small piece of butter, heaping teaspoonful baking powder, milk to make a thin batter. Cover the bottom of a buttered dish with some of the batter, then a layer of any fruit, alternating with batter, the batter being last. Steam an hour, and serve with any sauce. Anna Lees.

---

*Corn Starch Cocoanut Pudding*—One pint rich milk, two tablespoonfuls corn starch, one-half cup of sugar, three eggs, salt, vanilla. Stir eggs, sugar and milk together, put on the stove and when it begins to boil add the corn starch dissolved in a little milk. Stir constantly for a few minutes, when it will become a smooth paste, then add half a grated cocoanut, put into a mold and set to cool. Serve with whipped cream. Mrs. King.

*Graham Pudding.*—One cup each of molasses, sweet milk and raisins, two cups Graham flour, one egg, a little salt, one teaspoonful soda in molasses. Steam two hours.

Mrs. A. K. Brewster.

---

*Apple Batter Pudding.*—One pint rich milk, two cups of flour, teaspoonful salt, one-fourth teaspoonful soda, four eggs. Place in a pudding dish eight apples, pared and cored, and pour over them the batter. Bake an hour, and eat with a sauce of butter and sugar beaten to a froth. Mrs. Carpenter.

---

*Baked Indian Pudding.*—Two cups Indian meal, two quarts milk, one cup chopped suet, one-half cup butter, one cup brown sugar, one cup raisins, two eggs, two tablespoonfuls flour, same quantity cinnamon, a little salt. Heat the milk, stir in the meal, and when cool, add other materials. Bake in a slow oven three or four hours. Mrs. Capt. H. H. Brown.

---

*Pudding Sauce.*—Beat thoroughly the whites of two eggs with one cup powdered sugar; heat one tablespoonful brandy, same quantity of butter and four tablespoonfuls of water together, when boiling, stir in the eggs and sugar, but not till ready to serve. Miss King.

---

*Plum Pudding.*—One pint each of stoned raisins, currants, suet, (chopped fine,) flour and bread crumbs, one cup molasses, two cups of brown sugar, one of milk, four eggs, one nutmeg, a teaspoonful cinnamon, candied orange, citron, a teaspoonful soda, mixed well together, and steamed four hours.

Mrs. P. Bennett.

---

*Roly Poly Pudding.*—Make a dough of a quart of flour, butter size of an egg, two teaspoonfuls baking powder, one of salt, milk to make soft dough, roll out, spread with jelly, or any kind of fruit, fresh or canned, fold together, pinching the edges so that the juice does not run out, steam one hour, or wrapped in a thin bag, boiled forty minutes.

---

*Steamed Pudding.*—One pint of flour, a little salt, two teaspoonfuls baking powder, milk to make a soft dough, stir in any fruit, steam one hour. Mrs. Adams.

---

*Sauce.*—One cup pulverized sugar, two tablespoonfuls butter stirred to a cream, and add one half cup of cream, drop by drop.

Miss L. Dresher.

---

*Apple Tapioca Pudding.*—To one half teacupful tapioca add one and one half pints cold water. Let it stand on the stove till cooked clear, stirring to prevent burning, remove, sweeten and flavor with wine and nutmeg; pour this into a dish in which have been placed six or eight apples, pared and cored, bake until the apples are done. Serve cold with cream.

Mrs. Harry Baldwin.

---

*Rice Pudding.*—One quart of milk, one cup rice. Pour boiling water over rice several times to make it swell. Sweeten to taste with white sugar. Add one cup raisins, a little butter, a little salt. Bake two hours. Mrs. C. H. Brown.

---

*Walnut Pudding.*—One cup chopped nuts, two of graham or whole wheat flour, one half cup molasses, one half teaspoonful soda, mixed with the flour, one cup sweet milk, a little salt; steam two and a half hours.

---

*Lemon Meringues.*—One cup sugar, one lemon, a piece ot butter the size of a walnut, one tablespoon corn starch, yolks of two eggs, one cup of boiling water. Rub butter and sugar together add the eggs, rind and juice of the lemon, bake like a custard pie. When done beat the white of the eggs, add two tablespoonfuls sugar, and spread on the pie and brown. After pouring boiling water on the corn starch let it cool before using.

Mrs. Humphrey.

---

*Orange Pudding.*—Boil one quart of milk in a farina boiler, stir in quickly the yolks of three eggs, well beaten, two tablespoonfuls sugar, same of corn starch dissolved in a little milk, one teaspoonful vanilla. When the custard is cool, pour it over six large oranges sliced, and placed in a pudding dish, cover the whole with a meringue of whites three eggs, one half cup sugar, flavor with vanilla, and brown with a heated shovel.

Mrs. W. A. Frisbie.

---

*Cream Pie.*—Boil a pint of milk, and while hot stir in one half cup sugar, one egg, one fourth cup flour, two tablespoonfuls milk. Flavor with lemon and pour on the crust which must have been baked before. Mrs. Wm. Deane, Norwood, Mass.

---

*Mock Mince Pie.*—Six crackers, two cups boiling water, poured over crackers, one cup raisins, one cup salt pork chopped very fine, one cup molasses, one cup sugar, three-fourths cup vinegar, spice to taste. Miss Bartlett.

---

*Annie's Lemon Pie.*—Beat thoroughly together yolks of three eggs, one grated lemon, one cup sugar, two thirds cup cold water, two tablespoonfuls corn starch, piece of butter size walnut, bake in a rich crust. After it is baked cover the top with meringue made with whites of three eggs well beaten with two tablespoonfuls pulverized sugar. Mrs. W. B. Raymond.

---

*Suet Pudding.*—One cupful each of molasses, milk, suet well chopped, and fruit, four cups flour two teaspoonfuls soda. Steam two or three hours.

---

*Sauce.*—Beat thoroughly together, one cup sugar one half cup butter, add one cup boiling water, one well beaten egg, flavor to taste. Mrs. A. K. Brewster.

---

*Tapioca Cream.*—Soak three tablespoonfuls tapioca two hours in water sufficient to cover it. Boil the milk, stir in the tapioca, and when it boils again, add the yolks of three eggs well beaten with one cup sugar. Stir for ten minutes. Remove from the stove add well beaten whites. Serve cold. Miss Perkins.

---

*Mince Meat.*—Mix well together three lbs., cooked lean beef, two lbs. suet, five lbs. apples, all chopped as fine as possible, three lbs. raisins, one half a citron chopped fine, three lbs. sugar, one heaping teaspoonful each of ginger, cinnamon, and nutmeg, a scant half teaspoonful cloves, same of allspice, one teaspoonful salt, juice of two lemons, one pint of water in which the peel of the lemons have boiled for three minutes, and into which have been stirred one tumbler current jelly and as much cider as is needed to moisten the meat, set over the fire till heated through.

Mrs. Collins.

---

*Blackberry Wine.*—Measure the berries and then bruise them. To one gallon add one quart of boiling water, let it stand twenty-four hours, stirring occasionally, strain into a cask. To every gallon add two pounds sugar. Cork tight and let it stand three months, it will then be ready for use. G. P. H.

---

*Dish of Snow.*—Add to a quart of cream the whites of three eggs well beaten, four tablespoonfuls of sweet wine, sugar to taste and a teaspoonful vanilla, beat to a stiff froth and serve in a deep glass dish. Mrs. Marvin.

---

*Cottage Cheese.*—Strain through a bag, a pan of well scalded clabbered sour milk until the clabber is quite dry. Work this well with the hands, moisten by adding a little butter, cream and plenty of suet, then make into cakes. Mrs. P. R. Smith.

---

*Lemon Pie.*—Beat well together juice and grated rind of two lemons, three cups of sugar, three tablespoonfuls melted butter, yolks of six eggs, adding the stiff whites just as it is put into the paste. Mrs. R. L. Ganter.

*Coffee.*—One third Mocha two two thirds Java, or all of either, to taste; but do not fancy that first class coffee can be made from any of the cheaper grades, for it will fail; and, do not adulterate, for that was done before it reached you. If a filter be used, this is the better Method: use to every quart of water, one half cup of ground coffee; if the coffee be boiled, pour the boiling water on the coffee, which is ground much coarser than for filtering, where the boiling water leeches through the coffee, using the same proportions as already given, and boil *only three or four minutes*, closely covered. Mrs. W. C. Jacobs.

*Chocolate.*—Six tablespoonfuls of grated chocolate to one pint each of milk and water. Rub the chocolate smooth with cold water, then pour on the boiling water, boil twenty minutes, add the milk and boil five minutes longer, stirring frequently. Sweeten to taste. Mrs. C. P. Humphery

*A Nice Dessert.*—Core one dozen good ripe apples, filling the vacancy with sugar and a small piece of butter, put them into a shollow pan, filled half full of boiling water and set into the oven. When the apples have cooked for an hour, pour the juice into a pan and add a half cup of sugar, boiling it till it is thick syrup. The apples are to be returned to the oven for another hour, or till they are thoroughly done. Then put into a dish and the syrup poured over them. Serve with a tablespoonful of cream made thus; to the stiff beaten whites of two eggs add slowly one half a cup of pulverized sugar, flavored with vanilla, poured over each apple. Mrs. Mabley.

*Dulce De Co Co.*—Boil together until a thick syrup, one lb. granulated sugar and one cup of water, then add one grated cocanut cook five minutes, stirring constantly. Take from the fire add the beaten yolks of four eggs, mix well, pour into a flat oval dish, set in the oven to brown, and serve cold. Eva Mably.

*Russian Cream.*—Make a boiled custard of one quart of milk, one cup of sugar, yolks of four eggs; remove from the stove, add one third box gelatine dissolved in one half pint of hot water, beaten whites of four eggs and teapoonsful of vanilla. Serve cold. Eva Mabley.

*Ambrosia.*—Six sweet oranges, peeled and sliced, one pine apple peeled and sliced, the core grated, one grated cocoanut. Alternate layers of the fruit and grated nut, sprinkling pulverized sugar over each layer. Mrs. Fannie C. Wager.

*Jellied Fruit.*—Put into a dish, in layers, two oranges, cut in pieces, three bananas, sliced, and one pint of shredded pineapple, and pour over this a jelly made of one half box of gelatine dissolved in one pint of water, one and one half cups sugar, with juice of two lemons and two oranges. Serve cold with whipped cream. Mrs. J. Boyd.

---

*Wine Jelly.*—Pour a pint of cold water on a box of gelatine, let it stand one or two hours, then add one and half pounds white sugar, juice of two oranges and two lemons, teacup sherry wine Pour over all one quart boiling water, then strain.

Mrs. N. P. Goodhue.

---

*Velvet Cream.*—Dissolve one half ounce of gelatine in a teacup of white wine (keeping it standing in warm water.) When dissolved add to one pint of cream sweetened to taste, the gelatine and juice of one large lemon, and pour into the mold, setting in a cool place, till served. N. S.

---

*Orange Sherbet.*—One tablespoonful gelatine soaked in half a cup of cold water until soft then pour over one half cup boiling water, add one cup cold water, one cup sugar, the juiceof six oranges, which will be one pint of juice. When the sugar is dissolved, strain, and freeze. Mrs. A. L. Conger.

---

*Pineapple Sherbet.*—One tablespoonful gelatine soaked in cold water, till soft, then pour over one fourth of a cup of boiling water add one pint of cold water, one pint of sugar, one grated pine apple, then freeze. Mrs. A. L. Conger.

---

*Apple Cream.*—Pare six large apples, stew and mash them to a pulp. When cold add whites of four eggs well beaten, four tablespoonfuls sugar, beat well and flavor to taste.

Mrs. A. L. Conger.

---

*Spanish Cream.*—One fourth box gelatine, one and one half pints of milk, three eggs, three fourths cup of sugar. Boil the milk, and add yolks of eggs and sugar well beaten, then gelatine, boiling five minutes. Then remove from the fire, add the whites beaten stiff, and set on the ice. Mrs. P. W. Leavitt.

---

*Cream.*—Whip stiff a pint of cream, then add the whites of three eggs beaten stiff, and mixed, one cup of sugar, flavored with a teaspoonful of almond. Pour into a glass dish and set on ice. Mrs. P. W. Leavitt.

---

*Pudding Sauce.*—Beat to a cream one cup of butter and one cup of sugar, flavor with nutmeg or vanilla; pour over this, slowly, boiling water, stirring constantly till it is the consistency of cream. Miss Ganter.

*Baked Apple Pudding.*—Five moderate sized apples, two tablespoonfuls finely chopped suet, three eggs, three tablespoonfuls of flour, one pint milk. Mix the flour to a smooth batter with the milk, and the eggs, well beaten, put into a buttered dish. Cut the apples in halves and lay them in the batter; shake the suet over the top, and grate over the whole a little nutmeg. Bake an hour, and when served cover with fine sugar.

Mrs. Alden.

---

*Wine Jelly.*—One pound sugar, one pint of wine, one and one half ounces gelatine, one lemon, one quart water. Put the water over the gelatine, keep warm till dissolved, put in a porcelain kettle with sugar, wine and lemon, sliced, and boil twenty minutes. Mrs. Mary McCurdy.

---

*Velvet Cream.*—One half ounce of gelatine dissolved in white wine, one pint of cream, juice of one large lemon. Sweeten the cream to your taste.

---

*Mountain Dew.*—Make a pudding of the yolks of three eggs, one pint of milk, four tablespoonfuls of rolled crackers and a little salt. When baked, cover the top with whites of three eggs beaten stiff with one cup pulverized sugar, flavored with lemon, and return to the oven five minutes. Mrs. Chas. H. Brown.

At all times will it pay to visit our store, as we always have special bargains in our various departments.

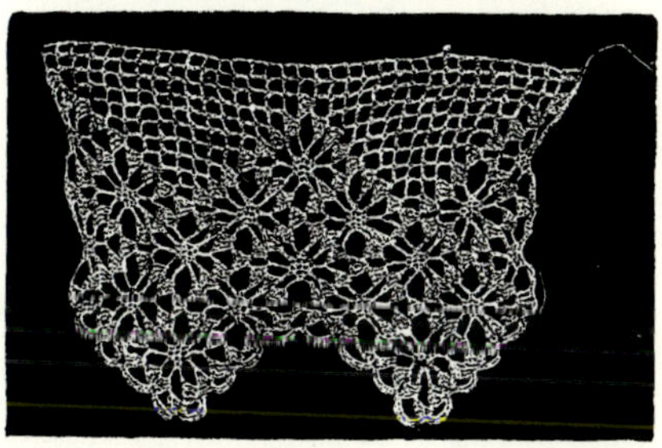

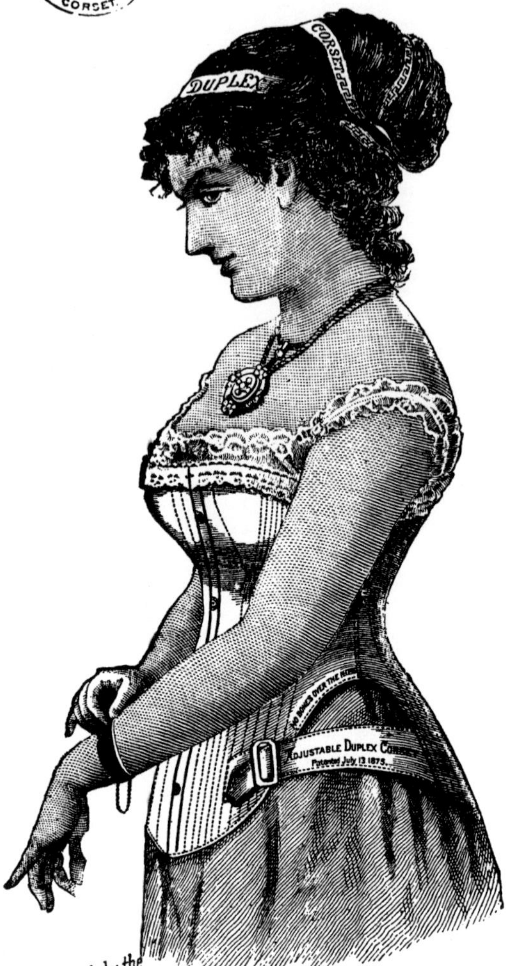
DUPLEX
CORSET
Adjustable Duplex Corset
Patented July 13 1875

# BREAD.

*Bread.*—Boil until soft, five moderate sized potatoes, mash and add two tablespoonfuls of flour. Pour in sufficient boiling water to make thickness of batter, stirring fifteen minutes, then add one quart of cold water. After cooling, add one cup strong yeast and let the mixture rise, in a warm place, six or eight hours. Then sufficient warm water to make five loaves, (one pint to a loaf; add flour to make a stiff batter, stirring well. Set it in a warm place to rise, and when light knead three quarters of an hour, and set again to rise. When light mold into loaves, put into pans, let rise and bake in a moderate ovan three-fourths of an hour. Mrs. Watters.

---

*Bread.*—Pare and slice three potatoes, cooking them in one quart of water till thoroughly done. While these are cooking put one cake fresh "compressed" yeast to soak in a teacup of warm water; as soon as soft stir in sifted flour to make a stiff bat ter, cover closely, setting in a basin of warm water. When the potatoes are done, mash them thoroughly, add a tablespoonful of salt and cold water to make a quart of liquid. When cool add the yeast, which, if good, will by this time have filled the bowl, and flour to make a stiff batter and set in a warm place, covering closely. When light, which should be in two hours, or less, knead till the dough will "cleave" from the board with sifted flour, being very careful not to use too much flour, and set to rise, covering with a flannel cloth. When light, in an hour, mold into loaves, put into pans, let them rise and bake in a moderate oven for forty-five minutes, or an hour. The bread should be out of the oven within five hours from its commecement. A.

---

*Rusk.*—One pint of milk, one cup yeast, one egg; stir in flour, as thick as for pancakes, and let it rise; then add one teacupful butter, one-half teacupful sugar, one-half teaspoonful soda, salt and flour to make a soft dough; when light work into biscuits, and when light bake. Miss Raff.

---

*Crumpets.*—One pint raised dough, three tablespoonfuls butter, three eggs, one-half cupful sugar. When the bread has passed its second rising, work in the melted butter, then eggs and sugar, beating together very light, mold into buscuits and bake twenty minutes. Mrs. Carpenter.

*Biscuit.*—Sufficient dough from the first kneading to make a medium sized loaf of bread. Beat together one egg and three tablespoonfuls of sugar, and add two ounces melted lard. Place this in a pan with the dough and knead till thoroughly mixed, without flour. Place on the kneading-board and work into a loaf, using as little flour as possible, and set to rise in a warm place; when light, mold into biscuits, which, after rising, must be baked in a moderate oven. Mrs. Watters.

---

*English Currant Bread.*—Three quarts of flour, one quart sweet milk, one pound currants, one pound raisins, seeded, two cupfulls sugar, one scant cupful butter, one-half cupful caraway seeds, four eggs, one-half cupful yeast, salt. Scald the milk, putting in the butter while warm, and when cool enough stir in the yeast, sugar, eggs and one quart of the flour. In the morning knead in the fruit and rest of the flour with caraway seeds, let it rise and make into four loaves, let them rise in the pans and bake an hour. Mrs. Wm. Robinson.

---

*Light Bread.*—Two quarts of scalded "Cerealine," eight tablespoonfuls of lard, six ounces of Fleischmann's yeast, eight quarts of flour, four teaspoonfuls salt; mix the wheat flour and "Cerealine" together; dissolve the salt in water, and dissolve six ounces of Fleischmann's yeast in a little cold water, and make into a stiff dough. Allow this mixture to raise about three hours, and then take out and make into six loaves of bread and set in a pan until it raises again, then about an hour in a hot oven.

---

*Griddle Cakes.*—Two cupfuls of scalded "Cerealine," one teaspoonful of sugar, two teaspoonfuls of baking powder, one and one-half cupfuls of milk, two cupfuls of flour, one teaspoonful of salt, one egg. Sift the flour, sugar, salt and baking powder together; add the "Cerealine" free from lumps, diluted with the beaten egg and milk; mix into a smooth batter; have the griddle well heated and greased; put the mixture on the griddle with a large spoon—about two spoonfuls to one cake; fry to a nice brown; turn carefully and fry as before, and serve with maple syrup.

---

*Parker House Rolls.*—At noon rub one large tablespoonful of lard into one quart of flour, make a hole in the center and set away. At night mix thoroughly a cup of yeast and a small half cup of sugar, with a pint of milk previously boiled and cooled, and a little salt, and pour this mixture into the hole in the flour. In the morning cut with a knife until all the flour is stirred in—not bread—and cut often during the day. About four o'clock P. M., roll out, cut, wash one half with melted butter, fold over, let them rise and bake in a quick oven. Mrs. Adams.

*Kentucky Biscuit.*—Make to a stiff dough one quart of flour, one pint of sweet milk, a piece of butter, size of an egg, a pinch of salt, and beat with rolling pin half an hour. Roll a quarter of inch thick, cut in small sizes and bake to a light brown.

Mrs. N. Monsarrat.

---

*Batter Bread or Egg Bread.*—One-half a cupful bread crumbs soaked in a pint of milk, two eggs, two cups of corn meal one tablespoonful butter, teaspoonful salt. Beat the eggs light, and the soaked crumbs to a smooth batter, stir in the melted butter and bake in shallow tins. Mrs. Carpenter.

---

*Corn Pone.*—One cupful of flour, two of corn meal, one pint of sweet milk, three eggs, one tablespoonful melted butter, two of sugar, one teaspoonful of soda and two of cream tartar, add a little salt. Mrs. Fannie C. Wager.

---

*Coffiee Bread.*—Bread dough, two tablespoonfuls of butter and lard, one teacup of sugar, a little salt. Roll out the dough not quite so thin as pie crust, spread butter on the layer, sprinkle with sugar and cinnamon, then roll and cut into biscuits: let them rise, and bake in a slow oven. Mrs. C. H. Brown.

---

*Corn Bread.*—Stir five pints of boiling water thick with corn meal, till it is well cooked; add a cup of brown sugar and a teaspoonful of salt. When cool add a pint of bread sponge and add flour to knead well, put in pans to rise, when light, bake in a moderate oven. C.

---

*Boston Brown Bread.*—One cup rye meal, one cup Indian meal, one cup of flour, one-half teaspoonful soda; sift all together, add one-half teacup molasses, a little salt, one-half pint milk, mix soft, and steam two hours. Miss Deane, Mass.

---

*Brown Bread.*—One-half pint sour cream, same quantity of milk and of sugar, one teaspoonful soda, one egg, salt, brown flour to make stiff that the batter will not run from the spoon.

Mrs. W. B. Raymond.

---

*Spider Corn Cake.*—Mix together one and two-thirds cups corn meal, one-third cup of flour, one-fourth of a cup of sugar, teaspoonful salt. Beat two eggs, add one cup sour milk and one of sweet, into which a small teaspoonful soda has been dissolved, pour the mixture upon the dry ingredients, and mix very thoroughly. Grease with butter a very hot frying pan, and pour the batter into it. Now pour in a cup sweet milk, *but do not stir the cake,* place in a hot oven and bake twenty or twenty-five minutes.

Mrs. Lincoln's Cooking School, Boston, Mass.

*Coffee Bread.*—Mix thoroughly into as much bread dough as will make a loaf to bake on a round pie tin, two tablespoonfuls butter and three of sugar. Let it rise, then roll into a sheet an inch thick. Put in a dripping pan to bake, letting it rise first, and bake in a quick oven. When done, take from the pan, spread over the top butter, and sprinkle with pulverized sugar and cinnamon, covering closely with the inverted pan.

H. N. A.

---

*Corn Meal Muffins.*—To one pint of meal add one cup of flour, butter, size of an egg, two well beaten eggs, one-half pint sweet milk, one-half cup fresh yeast. Mix at night; in the morning, bake in muffin rings.

---

*Flour Gems.*—One quart sour milk, one teaspoouful salt, one teaspoonful soda, butter, size of a hickory nut, two eggs, three teacups white flour. Mrs. W. B. Raymond.

---

*Graham Muffins.*—Two eggs, one-half cup molasses, one and a half cups graham flour, same quantity white flour, one teaspoonful each of soda and salt, one quart sour milk.

Mrs. W. B. Raymond.

---

*Brown Bread.*—Mix three small cups corn meal, two of graham flour, one large cup of sour milk, or cold water, one of molasses, one teaspoonful soda, one of salt, steam three hours, and brown fifteen minutes. Mrs. Frank Adams.

---

*Graham Bread.*—Mix two cups of buttermilk with one cup white flour, one-half cup molasses, in which a teaspoonful of soda has been stirred, a little salt and two and a quarter cups of graham flour. Mrs. McCurdy.

---

*Graham Wafers.*—Put a pinch of salt into one-half a pound of graham flour, wet it with one-half pint sweet cream, mixing quickly and thoroughly, roll as thin as possible, cut in strips, bake in a quick oven. Mrs. Harter.

---

*Corn Pone.*—One cup of flour, two cups of corn meal, (the white meal,) one pint of sweet milk, three eggs, three teaspoonfuls baking powder, one tablespoonful melted butter, two tablespoonfuls sugar and a little salt. Mrs. Fannie C. Wager.

---

*Potato Yeast.*—Boil a small handful of hops in a quart of water, strain on three good sized potatoes, grated, let it boil once, then add one-half cup of sugar, same quantity of salt, and when cool, one cake compressed yeast dissolved in lukewarm water.

Mrs. W. J. Ellis.

*Puff Cake.*—One pint of flour, pint sweet milk, two eggs, well beaten, small piece of butter, melted. Bake quickly in hot muffin irons. Mrs. Latham.

---

*Pan Perdu.*—Cut stale bread into pretty shapes, dipping into batter of egg and flour, fry in butter to a light brown. Sprinkle with sugar and cinnamon. Miss Carpenter.

---

*Rice Muffins.*—Beat hard together one cup cold boiled rice, one pint of flour, two eggs, one pint sweet milk and a little salt. Bake quickly. Mrs. N. Monsarrat.

---

*Egg Toast.*—Cut into inch squares four slices of bread, toasted to a light brown, buttering both sides, and put in a covered dish and keep hot. Beat six eggs and add one pint of sweet milk. Set in a kettle of boiling water a pan in which is one-half ounce of butter; when melted, add eggs and milk with salt and pepper to taste, stirring constantly, until the consistency of thick cream. Pour over the toast and serve hot. Angie Watters.

---

*Indian Bread.*—One pint sour milk, one cup molasses one teaspoonful of soda, two eggs, salt to taste; stir thick as cake, taking a large spoonful of shorts and corn meal alternately. Steam three hours. Mrs. H. H. Brown.

---

*Johnny Cake.*—One half cup sugar, same of shortening, two thirds cup sweet milk, two eggs, one cup corn meal, one of flour, two teaspoonfuls baking powder a little salt.

Mrs. E. W. Shook.

---

*Corn Bread.*—Two eggs, butter size of an egg, one cup milk, one teaspoonful salt, two tablespoonfuls sugar, one cup corn meal, one of flour, two teaspoonfuls baking powder. Mrs. M.

---

*Graham Bread.*—Mix to a stiff batter one quart sifted Graham meal, a pinch of salt, three teaspoonfuls baking powder mixed with flour, two tablespoonfuls of sugar, milk to make the batter. An egg beaten is an improvement. Bake in a moderate oven.

Mrs. W. Pardee.

---

*Shrove Tuesday Pancakes.*—One pint sweet milk, two eggs, flour to make a thin batter, a little salt. Fry in hot lard, sprinkle on each sugar and jelly, and eat hot. Mrs. Boyd.

---

*Scotch Short Bread.*—Three large cups of flour, one cup of butter, one half cup sugar. Knead all together and roll about three fourths of an inch thick, cut in squares and bake in a moderate oven. Mrs. Boyd.

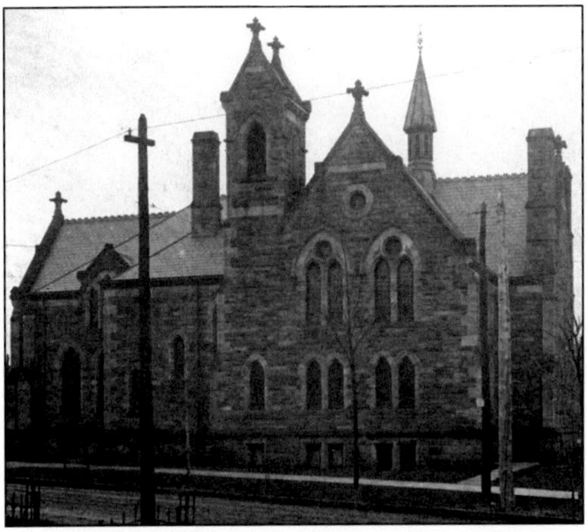

View of St. Paul's Church taken in 1891. The church was located on a triangular property bounded by East Market, Forge, and Fir Streets.

*From the Samuel Lane Collection. Courtesy of the Akron-Summit County Library.*

**Advertisement page 4.** The Burrows Bros. store has long been an institution in Cleveland. The business was founded in November, 1872, in the dark days following the panic, by Charles W. Burrows, a West Point graduate . . . and his younger brother, H. B. Burrows. The two brothers and a lone boy-of-all-work constituted the original staff of the store that opened at No. 7 Euclid Avenue on that rainy Saturday. The business grew steadily and in 1880 removed to larger quarters at 324 Euclid Avenue. . . . The Burrows Bros. Co. has long been known as one of the "high spots" in the bookselling business of the country. It is said that the present difficulties are expected to be temporary, being largely due to the opening of the new store and the frequent movings which the changes of recent years have necessitated. *Publishers Weekly*, 1917

**Advertisement page 10.** Back in 1863, when N. O. Stone established a one room store in lower Superior Avenue, Cleveland was a small city. . . . he knew the shoe business and as the city grew in wealth and population his

An 1890 view of Euclid Avenue showing a horse and buggy, a horse-drawn carriage and the Burrows Brothers Company which is located in the second building on the left side of the street.

*Courtesy the Cleveland Public Library, Photograph Collection*

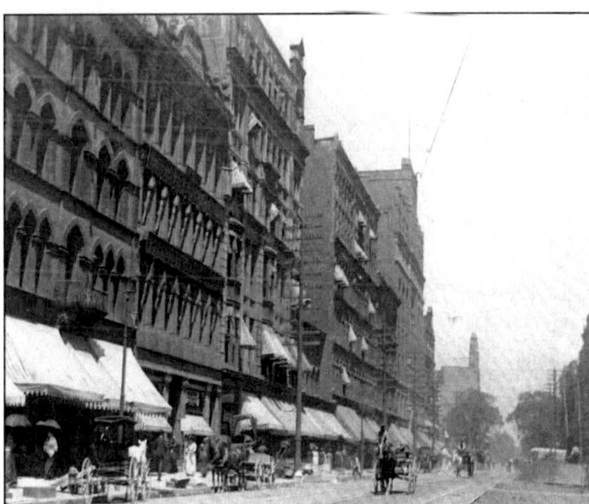

An 1889 view of a commercial section of Euclid Avenue just east of E. 4th Street showing the N. O. Stone & Company (on the left) and the Savings and Trust Company (on the corner).

*Courtesy the Cleveland Public Library, Photograph Collection.*

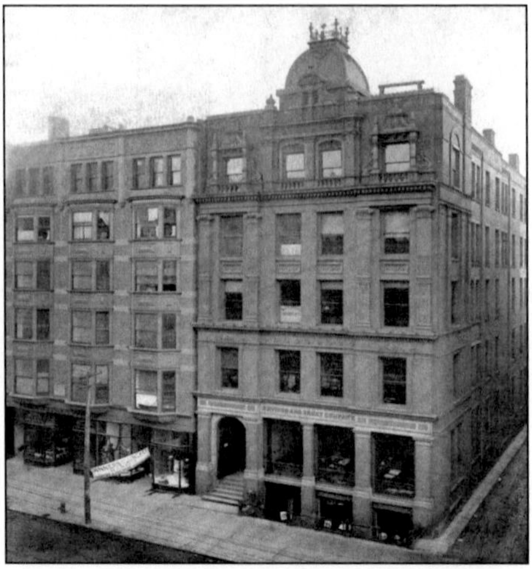

stock kept pace with the community developments. Today Cleveland is a city of nearly a million population. That one room store which Stone established has grown into three stores, all of them busy and prosperous. The down town store of the Stone Shoe Company which is on Euclid Avenue is one of the largest and finest stores in the country. Few stores in the country do as large a business annually. Three large floors are required to take care of the thousands of customers who visit this store daily. Mr. Stone lived to see a remarkable growth in his company. He died in December, 1912. *Boot and Shoe Recorder*, 1922

**Advertisement page 15.** The following letter, just received by the Imperial Granum Company from the publisher of one of the most influential of American medical journals, must certainly be most satisfactory to the manufacturers of that sterling food preparation: "Beginning with the grip, I ended up with a severe attack of gastric fever. This gave me an excellent opportunity to test Imperial Granum, and I assure you it was a great pleasure to have something that was at once so pleasant to the taste, so nourishing and so grateful to a delicate stomach. After being compelled to abstain from food for three or four days, I partook of the Imperial Granum quite freely, without the least disturbance of the stomach. As we have had much experience in dealing with delicate and sensitive stomachs, we thought it very remarkable that any food should prove so nourishing and yet could be taken so freely under such circumstances. I was glad to have such an opportunity to test your food, and I shall always be glad to recommend it." *The Alabama Medical and Surgical Age,* 1896.

**Advertisement page 18.** David L. King, the subject of this sketch, was born at Warren, Ohio, December 24, 1825, and graduated from Harvard College. He was admitted to the bar in 1848, and located at the City of Cleveland in 1851, but four years later removed to Akron, Ohio, at which city he made his home during his entire life . . . he was one of the active spirits in the promotion of the social and business interests of Akron. He was for many years identified with the Akron Sewer Pipe Company and other enterprises, was one of the original promoters of the Valley Railway, being at one time its President, and latterly organized the King Varnish Company. *Proceedings of the Scottish Rite (Masonic order),* 1901.

**Advertisement page 27.** Major E. Steinbacher died in Akron, Ohio, April 27th, of uraemic poisoning, having been ill since the first of the year, at the advanced age of seventy-eight years . . . He join[ed] the forty-niners, going overland to California in search of gold. Returning well compensated in 1851, he embarked in the drug and grocery business in the building where his business is now located, carrying on an extensive wholesale business. *Interstate Druggist, 1903*

**Advertisement page 28.** David Raymond Paige of Akron was born in Madison, Lake County, April 8, 1844. He graduated from Union college, Schenectady, New York, in 1865. He located in Akron, where he became a successful hardware merchant. He was treasurer of Summit County for four years, from 1875 to 1879. He was elected to the Forty-eighth congress in 1882 from the Twentieth district, composed of Summit, Wayne, Medina and a part of Cuyahoga, as a Democrat, notwithstanding the district was Republican by a large normal majority. He served one term. *Ohio in Congress,* 1901

**Advertisement page 29.** On July 16, the Board was informed of a strike at the works of Taplin, Rice & Co., located at Akron. . . . while the stove foundry of the concern was closed, the company demanded a reduction in the price formerly paid to molders in that department . . . and therefore the molders refused to accept the proposed reduction . . . The strike lasted three weeks and involved 30 men. *Annual Report of State Board of Arbitration,* 1897.

**Advertisement page 40.** [Samuel H. Halle] recognized an opportunity, and with his brother, Salmon P. Halle, purchased from the estate of Capt. T. S. Paddock the hat and fur shop located at 226 Superior Street. The firm of Halle Brothers continued at that location for a matter of three years, but at the end of that time found that under their aggressive management the business had outgrown the store . . . they moved to larger quarters at 89 Euclid Avenue. *A History of Cleveland and Its Environs,* 1918.

**Advertisement page 40.** The dentifrice known in Germany by this name [kalodont] is made by dissolving neutral soap in glycerin and rubbing with a suitable tooth powder, the proportions being adjusted to produce a soft mass. Carmine is used as a coloring, and the flavor may be given by adding sufficient of a mixture of

- Oil of peppermint 25 parts.
- Oil of lemon 6 parts.
- Oil of orris root 1 part.
- Oil of sage 1 part.

The preparation is usually put up in collapsible tubes. *Secret Nostrums and Systems of Medicine,* 1896.

**Advertisement page 47.** Weary & Kramer of Akron, Ohio—Originators of the "Akron" plan for churches allowing for the church auditorium and the Sunday-school hall to be united into one space. His designs included:

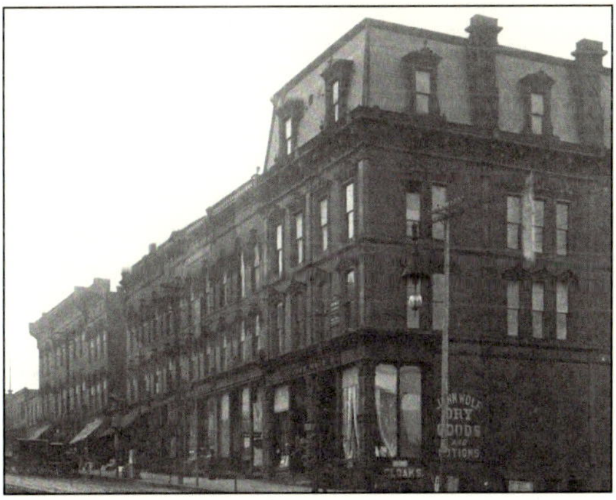

A view of the south side of Market Street from Main to High in 1891. John Wolf opened his dry goods store on the corner in 1875.

*From the Samuel Lane Collection. Courtesy of the Akron-Summit County Library.*

- Williamsbridge Methodist Episcopal Church (1893), Bronx, New York
- Arlington Avenue Presbyterian Church (1893), East Orange, New Jersey
- First Methodist Episcopal Church (1883), Canton, Ohio
- Hancock County Courthouse (1885), Findlay, Ohio
- Baldwin Cottage, Talcott Hall and Peters Hall, Oberlin College (1885-1887), Oberlin, Ohio

**Advertisement page 48.** Duryea's Satin Gloss Starch. Gives a glossy finish and renders fabrics durable. Is easily used, is economical and certainly the best article of the kind. *Handbook for the Kitchen and Housekeeper's Guide,* 1910

**Advertisement page 49.** P. L. Miles, Manufacturing Jeweler—Coming from Detroit in 1874, Mr. Miles opened out at No. 314 Euclid Avenue, the above named business . . . The departments of his business are designated as follows: manufacturing, engraving and designing, repairing and salesroom. He occupies the second and third floors of Lafayette block, containing five large rooms, in which are employed fourteen of the most skilled mechanics that can be found . . . This is the only jewelry manufactory in the city, employing more men and turning out more work by far than any other in the State. *Industries of Cleveland,* 1879

**Advertisement page 51.** White Sewing Machine Company—It was about 1876 that the White Sewing Machine Company manufactured its first sewing machine. The industry was started and was owned by the late Mr. Thomas H. White. Since that year, in a total of four decades, this company has manufactured and sold approximately 4,000,000 sewing machines. *A History of Cleveland and Its Environs,* 1918.

**Advertisement page 52.** White Marseilles (Castile soap)—White Castile soap is now made in almost all countries, and generally with the artificial sodas, and even in Marseilles these sodas are now being used. Yet in some factories the barilla is still used as the base; this alkali, containing a certain percentage of potash, gives a plastic consistency to the soap which has added to its popularity. This effect is now usually produced by the addition of a drying oil, such as hempseed, sesame, ground-nut, poppy or

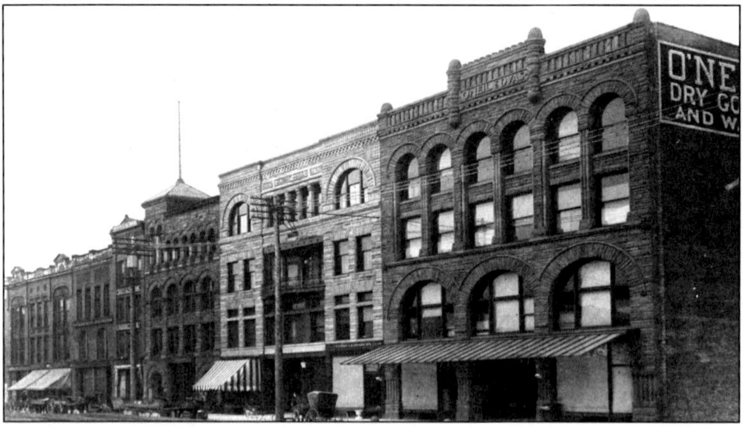


A view of the west side of Main Street from Mill to Market. On the right is the O'Neil & Dyas dry goods store. O'Neil and Dyas opened their first store at 114 East Market Street in 1877. They moved to this building in 1889. *From the Samuel Lane Collection. Courtesy of the Akron-Summit County Library.*

cotton seed oil to the amount of 15 to 25 per cent, of the olive oil. *A Technical Treatise on Soap and Candles,* 1881.

**Advertisement page 56.** Frank Dowd began practice in Jamestown, N. Y., 1882, where he invented, and practically used the first fixed bridge- work done in that place . . . he came here [Akron, Ohio] and practiced crown and bridge-work, and taught dentistry to his wife M. A. Dowd; son H. H. Dowd; present wife K. H. Dowd; brother J. C. Dowd . . . In 1885 he invented an all-cord, suspension dental engine . . . In 1911 he devised a set of instruments for attaching crowns to roots so that the pin will not bend and permit an open joint between the crown and root . . . His patent safety device consists of buffers which arise from the track and prevent cars from passing by them. This device was accepted by the City R. R. Co. In 1911 he patented a vehicle wheel, which consists of a series of spiral springs within the rubber tire; this takes the place of the pneumatic tire on automobiles, as a puncture at any place will not affect the working of the wheel. *History of Dentistry in Cleveland, Ohio,* 1911.

**Advertisement page 57.** [T]he Barber Match Company of Akron, Ohio [was] established in 1847. This factory is the largest in the country, if not in the world, having a capacity of 100,000,000 matches per day. Other factories also started in the East and West. In 1881, 29 of these were incorporated as the Diamond Match Company, a corporation which has grown to be one of the most successful manufacturing enterprises on the continent. It has a capital of $6,000,000, upon which dividends are regularly paid . . . The Diamond Match Company consumes 27,000,000 feet of pine lumber in the manufacture of matches annually, and 20 tons of paper and straw-board a day, all of which it manufactures. It has a tract of white pine in nearly one body of 400,000,000 feet, enough for many years' supply. *King's Handbook of the United States,* 1992.

**Advertisement page 59.** The superfine quality of cereal products is a credit to the enterprise of American manufacturers . . . These and other goods in that line are extensively manufactured by the F. Schumacher Milling Company, of Akron, Ohio, its president, Ferdinand Schumacher, now commonly known as The Oatmeal King, being the pioneer oat-meal manufacturer of the United States. He began on a small scale in 1856, and, gradually increasing his facilities, lost half a million dollars by a destructive fire on the morning of March 6, 1886. Nothing daunted, he immediately

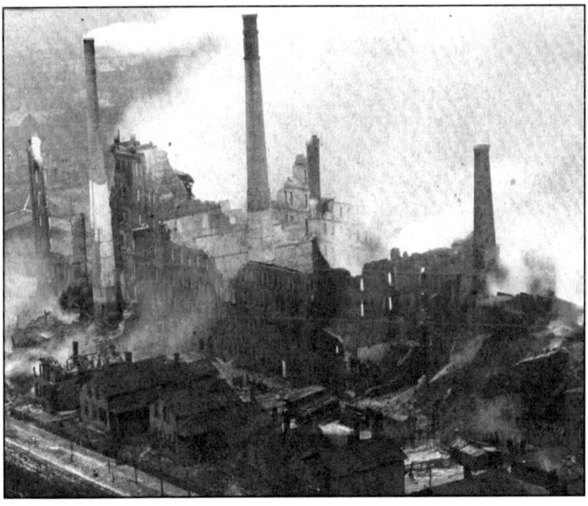

Fire at the Schumacher Mills that started on March 6, 1886, lasted two days, and destroyed every building except the Empire Mill and a new office.

*From the Samuel Lane Collection. Courtesy of the Akron-Summit County Library.*

chartered a company with an authorized capital of $2,000,000. The plant consists of five mills, converting daily 14,000 bushels of wheat, oats, corn, barley, rye, and buckwheat into choice food for man and beast . . . Running night and day, the firm employs 300 men and 70 girls, putting up cereals in one and two pound packages. The annual output amounts to $3,000,000. *King's Handbook of the United States,* 1892.

**Advertisement page 60.** The origins of the Akron Greek community date to the closing decades of the nineteenth century. It is believed that the first Greek settler was Nick Laskaris, who moved to Akron, Ohio, from Elmira, New York, in 1880 . . . By 1897, Laskaris owned a retail and wholesale fruit store at 160 South Howard Street. The area around Howard Street attracted additional numbers of early Greek immigrants and with time it evolved into a Greek residential cluster. Later, several coffeehouses and other ethnic establishments located in this area. *GeoJournal*, Vol. 69, No. 2-3, 2007.

**Advertisement page 61.** Among the industries of East Dover Hundred is the Richardson & Robbins canning factory of Dover, the excellence of whose products have won international approval. In 1856 the canning business was started in earnest, and that year six hundred cans were put on the market. The excellence of the output created such a demand that it was found necessary to increase the business, and a larger building was purchased. In 1862 the output had grown to 40,000 cans, and a still larger building was required. *History of the State of Delaware,* 1908.

**Advertisement page 74.** The improved mowing, reaping, and binding machines of to-day cut the grass and grain upon these immense fields; and the most important part of these machines is the cutting apparatus, the mower knives, serrated sickles and sections, the manufacture of which is carried on as a specialty. The largest manufacturer of these goods in the United States, or in the world, is the Whitman & Barnes Manufacturing Company, of Akron, O., and Syracuse, N. Y. The company was incorporated in 1877, with a capital of $400,000; but to meet the wants of their business this capital has since been increased to $2,000,000 . . . In addition to manufacturing knives, sickles, and sections, they are the largest manufacturers of spring cotters in the world, and make many specialties and repairs. *King's Handbook of the United States,* 1892.

**Advertisement page 75.** The name of Barbour has been associated with the spinning of flax for many long years... Two of the four brothers accordingly came to these shores to look the field over. They decided on Paterson as the seat of their future energies and in 1864 purchased a mill which had been used for some years by John Colt in the manufacture of cotton . . . The Barbours had the brains and the energy, the market was ready for them and so all that remained was manufacturing and exploitation. The two brothers who established the industry in this country were Thomas and Robert . . . Thomas attended to the business end of the proposition and soon became a commanding figure in commerce in the metropolis. Robert spent most of his time in Paterson, looking after the manufacturing. Robert died on March 24, 1892, and ten years later, on March 25, Thomas followed his brother to the grave. *History of Paterson and Its Environs,* 1920.

**Advertisement page 76.** The "Bortree Manufacturing Company" is engaged in the manufacture of corsets and hoop skirts. It is one of the largest manufacturers of this class of goods in this country. Most of its work is after patents owned by Mr. Bortree of the company. Constant employment is given to some 200 girls, besides other employes. *Michigan Historical Collections*, 1880.

**Advertisement page 77.** Mr. Herbert P. Hitchcock, insurance agent at Akron, O., died last Saturday from blood poisoning caused by the slip of a razor while cutting a corn. He was fifty-two years old. *The Weekly Underwriter,* 1894.

**Advertisement page 83.** No impure or injurious article is used in the manufacture of the Atlantic & Pacific Tea Co.'s baking

powder. Pure cream of tartar and pure bicarbonate of soda are used in the manufacture of the Atlantic & Pacific Tea Co.'s baking powder.
There is no secret about the formula of the Atlantic & Pacific Tea Co.'s baking powder. Anyone can make it just as good as they; but the trouble is that many of the baking powders put on the market are compounded of an inferior quality of commercial chemicals. *Cleveland Medical Gazette,* 1888.

**Advertisement page 84.** Union Porcelain Works, Brooklyn.—This is the only manufactory in the United States making a true hard porcelain. Originally established about 1854 by a number of German workmen as a manufactory of bone china, it was rescued from extinction, which their want of knowledge and dishonesty nearly precipitated, by Mr. Thos. C. Smith, who had joined them in 1857 . . . It was not, however, until 1865 that he was able to place on the market plain white tableware. In the year following he commenced to decorate, his chief designer and modeler being Karl Muller, who has produced several important pieces, such as the Century and Keramos vases. Vases and statuettes are made, but the principal production is tableware, which is of excellent quality, both in body and glaze, and, on the whole, tastefully decorated. *The Encyclopedia of Ceramics,* 1902

**Advertisement page 85.** This branch of [starch] manufacture is carried on, on a large scale, by Julius J. Woods & Co.; established in 1843. The capacity of their factory is to work up five hundred bushels of corn per day, employing a capital of $100,000 and forty hands. *Columbus, Ohio: Its History, Resources, and Progress,* 1873.

**Advertisement page 102.** Cerealine is a product made from Indian corn . . . The corn is first thoroughly cleaned in the dry state. It is then steamed just enough to soften and toughen the germs and husks, so that they may not grind up in the reduction which follows, while the glutinous or starchy interior remains practically unaffected by the steam. The corn thus steamed is immediately coarsely ground or broken, preferably between corrugated rolls, reducing it to a coarse meal composed of separate hulls, germs, and granules of the starchy portion mixed with some little finely-reduced starchy meal. This material is at once screened to separate therefrom the hulls as well as the fine meal. The remaining material, composed of coarse starchy granules and germs, is then sized into grades by means of suitable screens or sieves, and then while the germs are still soft, submitted, each grade separately, to the action of a mechanical picker or germ extractor for picking or extracting the soft germs from the harder, coarse starchy granules. This cleansed granular material is then again steamed to soften it, and is finally, while still soft pressed and dried, preferably by passing it through hot rolls, so that the granules will be flattened into thin hard flakes, which constitute the cerealine. *American Chemical Review,* 1885.

**Advertisement page 103.** About this time a request came to Mr. Smith from Mr. Seaman desiring him to come to Cleveland, where Mr. Seaman was then in business. In 1836 he complied with the request, and after a brief conference became the partner of Mr. Seaman in the shoe business. Thus, without one written line of partnership articles, the firm of Seaman & Smith began, and it continued without jar or variance until the death of Mr. Seaman in 1877, a period of more than forty years. This was the longest partnership connection without change until then known in Cleveland. *Annals of the Early Settlers Association of Cuyahoga County,* 1887.

**Advertisement page 104.** Messrs. Decker & Wilbur have recently fitted up a parlor studio among the palaces of Euclid Avenue, and have a most complete and cozy place of business. Their work is in harmony therewith, and surely they should be both prosperous and happy in such a model atelier. *Photographic Times and American Photographer,* 1883.

**Advertisement page 129.** David Thomas . . . was born at Millersburg, O., March 9, 1841, the son of George and Jane (Wilson) Thomas. David Thomas was educated in the public schools of Akron . . . At the close of the [Civil] war he returned to Akron, and in partnership with his father, engaged in the lumber and planing-mill business, which he built up until it has reached large proportions, and until 100 men are employed by the Thomas Lumber & Building Co., of which Mr. Thomas is president. *The National Cyclopaedia of American Biography,* 1895.

**Advertisement page 130.** With an order for 1 doz. Alexander's Liver and Kidney Tonic, or a regular 3-doz. case at $8.00 per doz., we will send, besides powders that go with each bottle, as many circulars as you can use, with your card as sole agent; hangers and display posters, paraffin signs, caps, transparencies, stickers, etc., making an elegant display. We give you a written contract authorizing you to refund the money if not satisfactory to your customers. *Meyer Brothers Druggist,* 1905.

**Advertisement page 130.** Jacob Snyder, Architect. His designs included:

- Ohio Agricultural College (1871), Columbus, Ohio
- Hower House (1871), Akron, Ohio
- Methodist Episcopal Church (1873-1875), Painesville, Ohio

**Advertisement page 131.** The McNeil Boiler Company, Akron, Ohio, manufacturer of Cook water tube boilers, has just completed two new buildings . . . and has placed contract for another building . . . This company's stockholders have recently voted to increase its capital stock from $100,000 to $150,000. *American Industries,* 1909.

**Advertisement page 132.** Dr. Price began manufacturing baking powder on Lake Street in Chicago, near Market street, and there continued for two years, when the great fire of 1871 destroyed his plant. Not discouraged by this loss, he again started in business at Nos. 47 and 49 Lake street, where he remained for two years . . . his trade demanded more commodious quarters and he removed to South Water street . . . He then removed to 108 and 110 Randolph Street for nine years after which time the Price Baking Powder Company building became a landmark in the manufacturing district, just north of the river at Dearborn avenue and Michigan street . . . Dr. Price had also begun the manufacture of flavoring extracts. Chemical investigation and experience and deep research along this line had given to the world in flavoring extracts that which is equal in quality to his baking powder, and this feature of his business has gradually assumed great prominence and added to his name new fame commensurate with that conferred upon him when his first discovery became known. His manufactures are in millions of homes throughout the land. *Chicago: Its History and Its Builders, a Century of Marvelous Growth,* 1912.

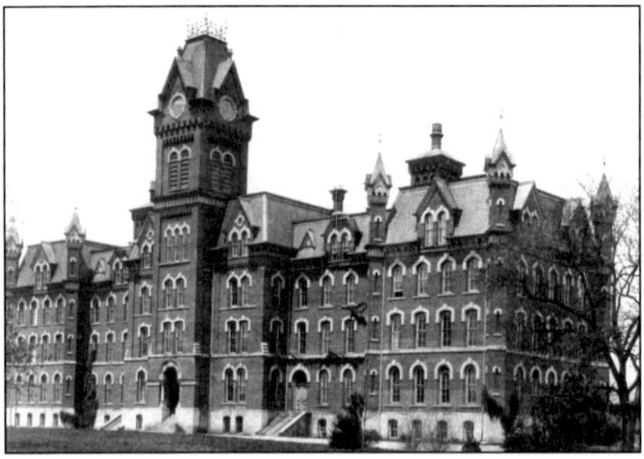

A view of the Ohio Agricultural and Mechanical College, 1881.

*Courtesy The Ohio State University Photo Archives.*

# Gate City Stone Filter Company

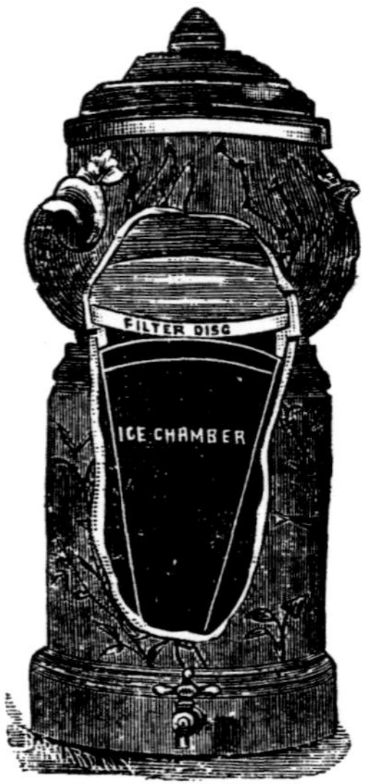


This open cut represents our China Filters with Filter Disc and **Patent Ice Chamber**. By this arrangement the filtered water is cooled without mingling with the ice.

**Manufactory and Depot at Union Porcelain Works,**

GREENPOINT, N. Y.

## Best Filter ever Invented !

---

**Cheap Stone Jar Filters for the Kitchen.**

FINE PORCELAIN (WITH ICE CHAMBERS)

For Dining-Rooms, Halls and Offices.

**LASTS A LIFETIME WITHOUT CHANGE.**

**No Metal Used.**—*All common metals generate poison* when in *contact* with *water. No Charcoal, Sand* or *other Compound* used. They *all absorb, retain* and become *foul with living organisms. Charcoal has no chemical effect on water.* Our Filtering Medium is a *natural stone.* No matter whether the impurities are organic or inorganic, they are left on the *surface of the stone*, which is as easily cleaned as an ordinary water-pail or pitcher.

**For Descriptive Price List address**

***Office and Salesroom, 839 Broadway and 65 E. 13th St.,***

**NEW YORK CITY.**

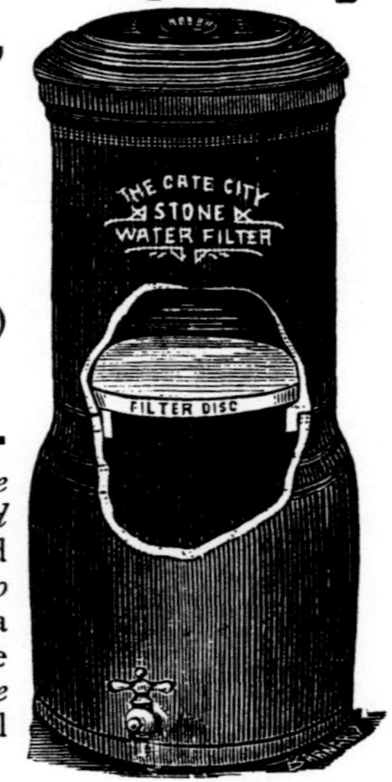


This open cut represents our Stoneware Filters in operation, showing the stone disc through which the water is filtered.

**The Stone Jar Filters have no Ice Chambers.**

# Some Facts About Starch and Its Use.

Ask for Wood's Columbus Corn Starch, the Purest and Best.

Wood's Gloss and Corn Starch, the Standard of Excellence.

Every housekeeper has at some time felt discontented because she cannot produce the highly polished linen turned out in steam laundries with the aid of machinery. She envies the immaculate work of the laundry, which she cannot imitate with ordinary starch. The inconvenience of sending the family washing to a public laundry, together with the expense attending it, deters many from doing so. The use of

## WOOD'S GLOSS POLISH STARCH

will enable every one without additional expense to finish at home laundry work equal to that of any steam laundry.

**THE ADVANTAGES OF WOOD'S GLOSS POLISH STARCH ARE:**

1st. Its simplicity. No expert required. Any housekeeper or servant can use it with the most satisfactory results.

2d. It not only stiffens and gives to linen a perfect gloss, but also makes a garment wear longer without soiling. The smooth surface it imparts resists dirt.

3d. It renders washing easier, as the Polish Wax fills the pores of the fabric so that dirt cannot penetrate. The Polish Wax has an affinity for soap, and immediately saponifies when brought into contact with soap and water; this loosens and expels the dirt without the vast amount of rubbing usually required in washing clothes.

4th. It is economical. It produces the best results at the expense of the least labor in both washing and ironing, and in so doing lessens the wear and tear.

5th. Its evident merit. The Laundress sees what she is using. That it stiffens, whitens, and gives a beautiful polish. It does not discolor or injure in the slightest degree the finest fabrics, but makes them wear longer without soiling, wash easier, iron easier; and thus last longer.

6th. It is inexpensive. A package of WOOD'S GLOSS POLISH STARCH, costing 10 cents at retail, contains one pound of finest Crystal Starch over 98 per cent pure, and a large cake of Polish Wax, so that buyers secure the cake of Polish with a pound of Starch for 10 cents, which is no more than is usually charged for some other brands of ordinary starch.

WOOD'S GLOSS POLISH STARCH is within the reach of all, and there is no reason why every Family should not have as finely finished linen as can be produced in any laundry.

**Ask Your Grocer for It. A Trial will Convince You of Its Merits. Be sure you get**

## WOOD'S GLOSS POLISH STARCH.

Manufactured by THE JULIUS J. WOOD STARCH CO., Columbus, O.

## CAKES.

*Angel Food.*—Whites of eleven eggs, one and one half cup of sifted granulated sugar, (the tumbler for measuring must hold two and one fourth gills,) one tumbler sifted flour, one teaspoonful each of vanilla and cream tartar. Sift the flour four times then add the cream tartar and sift again, but measure it before putting in the cream tartar, and sift the sugar before measuring. Beat the eggs to a stiff froth on a large platter; on the same platter add the sugar very lightly, then the flour, in the same manner, lastly the vanilla. Do not stop beating until it is put into the pan to bake, bake forty minutes in a moderate oven, try with a straw, and if it seems too soft let it remain in the oven a few minutes longer. Do not open the oven till the cake has been in fifteen minutes. When done, turn the pan upside down to cool, and when cold loosen the sides from the pan with a sharp knife, then ice. Use the pan made for baking that cake, as it has feet, and use no butter or paper in the pan. Miss H. Lansing.

*Angel Food.*—Whites of eleven eggs, one and one half cups granulated sugar, one coffecup flour, one teaspoonful cream tartar, one-half teaspoonful of vanilla, and a pinch of salt. Sift the flour three times before, and six times after putting in the cream tartar. Beat the eggs to a stiff froth, having previously put in the salt. Add the sugar very lightly to the eggs, then the flour in the same manner and, lastly, the vanilla, mixing all as quickly as poosible after the eggs are beaten—use only the egg beater. Turn immediately into a round tin with a funnel in the center—use neither butter or paper the tin—and bake in a moderate oven slowly for about an hour. When done (try with a straw) turn the tin upside down on the edge of two cups, being very careful that the cups do not touch the cake. When cool, loosen from the pan with a sharp knife. The oven should not be opened until the cake has been in ten minutes. Slow mixing or quick baking spoils the cake. Mrs. H. H. Brown.

*Almond Cake.*—Two cupfuls of flour, two of sugar, six tablespoonfuls melted butter, five eggs. beaten separately, three-fourths cup milk, two heaping teaspoonfuls baking powder. Bake in layers and put together with the following; one pint milk two eggs, a small piece of butter, one tablespoonful corn starch. Heat the milk to nearly boiling, and add the starch previously dissolved in milk, then add the eggs well beaten with three heaping tablespoonfuls white sugar. Let it come to a boil stirring constantly. When cold flavor with vanilla and almond. Blanch one half pound of almonds, chop fine and add to the above. Ice the top and sides of the cake heavily, and garnish the edge of the top layer with blanched almonds. Mrs. E. O. Stanley.

*Mrs. Madison's Whim.*—Two pounds each of flour butter and sugar; beat the butter to a cream. Beat the yolks of twelve eggs with the sugar, the whites to a froth; two wine glasses of rose water in which lemon rinds have been steeped, one nutmeg, grated, one teaspoonful soda dissolved in hot water. Beat well together, add two pounds raisins, stoned and chopped, and a little citron cut into small pieces. It will keep three months.

Mrs. R. H. Wright.

*Angel Cake.*—Whites of ten eggs, one-half cup sugar, one cup flour, a little salt, one teaspoonful cream tarter. Mix all the ingredients very thoroughly, except the eggs, adding the beaten whites last. Mrs. A. K. Brewster.

*White Loaf Cake.*—The whites of seven eggs, two cups of sugar. one small cup of butter, one and one-half cups of milk, two teaspoonfuls baking powder, two cups of raisins boiled soft rolled in flour, three cups of flour. Mrs. Adams.

*Loaf Cake.*—Three cups light bread dough, two cups sugar, one of butter, three eggs, one nutmeg, one teaspoonful cinnamon, two teaspoonfuls baking powder stirred in the last thing before putting the cake into the oven. Raisins to taste. Mrs. W. F.

*Empire Cake.*—Stir to a cream one-half cup butter, one and one-third cups sugar, add whites of three eggs, two-thirds cup sweet milk, two of flour, two-thirds of a cup of raisins stewed soft, two teaspoonfuls baking powder, flavoring with lemon.

Mrs. E. Dodge.

*Boiled Icing.*—Boil one pound sugar with a little water, until it will "thread" when dropping from the spoon; then take from the fire and while it is boiling hot, add the whites of three eggs very well beaten, stirring them into the syrup as rapidly as possible.

Mrs. W. C. Jacobs.

*Coffee Cake.*—Bread dough, two tablespoonfuls butter and lard mixed. one teacup sugar, a little salt. Roll out not quite so thin as pie crust; spread butter on the layer, and sprinkle white sugar and cinnamon then roll and cut into biscuits. Let them rise and bake in a slow oven. Mrs. C. H. Brown.

*Lemon Cake.*—One cup butter, three of sugar, four of flour, one of milk, five eggs, one teaspoonful soda, one lemon, grated.
Miss Carpenter.

---

*Hickory Nut Cake.*—One pound sugar, one-half pound butter, one pound flour, one cup milk, four eggs, one cup boiled raisins, one large bowl chopped nut meats, two teaspoonfuls baking powder. Mrs. Merrill.

---

*Mother Cobb's Loaf Cake.*—One cup butter, two cups sugar, three cups dough as it is ready for the pans, four eggs. Spices, one teaspoonful of each, one cup raisins, half cup currants, add one teaspoonful of soda, just before you stop stirring. Put all in an earthen dish, and mix thoroughly with the hand for twenty minutes. Do not add any more flour, the dough is sufficient. This quantity makes two cakes. Bake immediately.
Mrs. J. M. Cobb.

---

*Sponge Cake.*—One and one half cups sugar, three eggs, two cups flour, one-half cup water, pinch of salt, two even teaspoonfuls baking powder. Mrs. Page.

---

*Date Cake.*—One-half cup butter, two of sugar, three of flour whites five eggs, two teaspoonfuls baking powder. Bake in layers and put together with boiled frosting, then boiled dates, one pound, cut in halves. Mrs. Alfred Brewster.

---

*White Cake.*—One and one-half cups sugar, one-half cup of butter, one-half cup of corn starch, three-fourths cup of milk, one of flour, two heaping teaspoonfuls of baking powder.
Mrs. C. E. Carter.

---

*Almond Sponge Cake.*—One pint sugar, same quantity of flour, one teaspoonful salt, whites of ten eggs, yolks of three, four tablespoonfuls water, one teaspoonful baking powder, one cup grated almonds. Beat sugar, water, almonds and yolks of eggs very thoroughly, then add half the flour, then half the beaten whites, then rest of the flour, finally rest of whites. Flavor with almond, and bake in small cakes. Miss Raff.

---

*Ice Cream Cake.*—Stir together one-half cup butter, and one and one-half cups sugar, add one and one-half cups flour, one-half cup corn starch, one-half cup sweet milk, whites six eggs two teaspoonfuls baking powder. Flavor to taste.
Mrs. J. H. Collins.

---

*Cocoanut Custard Cake.*—One and one-half cups sugar, one-half cup water, four eggs, two cups of flour, three teaspoonfuls baking powder. Beat together the sugar and yolks of eggs then add water and flour, and lastly the whites whipped to a stiff froth Bake in three layers, and put together with a custard, made of one cup sweet milk, two tablespoonfuls sugar, one tablespoonful corn starch, two tablespoonfuls cocoanut, the yolk of one egg, reserving the white for frosting the top of the cake.

Mrs. W. A. Caldwell.

---

*Harrison Cake.*—Four eggs, one and one-half cup molasses same quantity brown sugar, one cup butter, one of coffee, or sour milk, five cups flour, two teaspoonfuls soda, one and one-half teaspoonfuls each of cinnamon and cloves, one nutmeg, one cup currants, and of seeded raisins. Mrs. W. J. Ellis.

---

*Sponge Cake.*—Beat separately yolks and whites of nine eggs, stir in the weight of eight eggs in flour, and of four in sugar, one lemon, grated. Mrs. W. B. Raymond.

---

*Hickory Nut Cake.*—One and one-half cups sugar, half cup butter, three fourths cup sweet milk, two cups flour in which is sifted two teaspoonfuls baking powder, whites four eggs beaten to a stiff froth. Bake in sheets. Icing and Filling:—Whites of three eggs beaten stiff, three large tablespoonfuls white sugar one cup chopped nut meats. Flavor with vanilla.

Mrs. A. K. Brewster.

---

*My Lady's Cake.*—Two cups powdered sugar, one half cup butter, one cup sweet milk, three cups flour, whites five eggs, two teaspoonfuls baking powder, flavor. Flora Sumner.

---

*White Face Cake.*—One-half cup butter, one and a half of sugar, two and one-fourth of flour, whites three eggs, two teaspoonfuls baking powder. Sara Buckingham.

---

*Loaf Cake.*—One pint of dough, one-half pint of butter, one pint of sugar, four eggs, one teaspoonful cinnamon, one-half teaspoonful soda, one nutmeg, raisins. Sara Buckingham.

---

*Almond Custard Cake.*—Six eggs, two cups sugar one cup butter, one cup sweet milk, two cups corn starch, two cups flour, two teaspoonfuls baking powder, flavor with vanilla and bake in jelly pans. Spread between the layers a custard made of one cup of thick sour cream mixed with a pound of blanched almonds beaten fine and sugar to make very sweet. Beat the yolks of two eggs until very light with sugar. Add to the cream with one or two tablespoonfuls of corn starch, flavoring with vanilla; then mix well with this the whites well beaten with sugar. The custard must be very sweet. Mrs. H. H. Brown.

*Fruit Cake.*—One pound each of flour, butter, sugar and citron; three pounds currants, two pounds raisins one-fourth pounds each of cinnamon, nutmeg and mace, ten eggs, one gill each of brandy and molasses, and a little soda. Mrs. Alden.

---

*Plain Cake.*—Beat one cup white sugar and yolks of three eggs to a froth, add one-half cup each of butter and sweet milk, then two cups of flour into which two teaspoonfuls baking powder has been sifted, lastly whites of three eggs and flavoring,

Mrs. Fay.

---

*Corn Starch Cake.*—Beat together the whites of six eggs, two cups pulverized sugar, one cup butter, one of corn starch, two, flour, two teaspoonfuls baking powder, one teaspoonful lemon. Bake in square tin. Miss Rose Day.

---

*Pound Cake.*—One pound each of butter, sugar, flour and eggs, one teaspoonful soda, two teaspoonfuls of cream tartar, one-half pound citron. Mrs. Alden.

---

*Harlequin Cake.*—One cup of butter, two cups of sugar, three of flour one cup of milk, whites of six eggs, three teapoonfuls baking powder. Bake in four pans, coloring one brown with chocolate, one pink, one salmon. Put the layers together with lemon custard. Mrs. F. S. Newton.

---

*Loaf Cake.*—Four cups of dough, three of light brown sugar, one and one-half cups of butter, four eggs one tablespoonful cinnamon, one nutmeg, beaten well together, allowed to rise and baked in two loaves.

---

*White Cocanut Cake.*—Four cups flour, three of sugar, one of butter, one of milk; whites of ten eggs, two teaspoonfuls baking powder, one-half grated coconut put into the cake, the other half with whites three eggs and one-half cup sugar make frosting.

Mrs. W. B. Raymond.

---

*Pound Cake.*—One pound of flour, one pound of sugar, three-fourths pound of butter, nine eggs, one nutmeg, three teaspoonfuls baking powder, one-half teaspoonful milk. H. B. R.

---

*Mrs. Carpenter's Wedding Cake.*—One and one-fourth pound butter, one pound flour, one pound sugar, whites of seven eggs, yolks of ten, two tablespoonfuls cinnamon, one of ginger, one of mace, two of nutmeg, one of cloves, one gill of brandy. Mix spices, brandy and large spoonful soda together. Beat the butter to a cream then add the sugar, and afterward beaten eggs, spices and flour. Bake in a brisk oven from three to four hours.

*Orange Cake.*—Two cups sugar, one-half cup butter, same quantity of cold water, three cups flour, two teaspoonfuls baking powder, one orange, grated, beat eggs separately. Spread between the layers frosting with grated orange stirred in.

Mrs. H. H. Brown.

---

*Cream Cakes.*—One half pint water, two-thirds cup butter; when boiling add one and a half cups flour. Cool and add five eggs, well beaten, and one-fourth teaspoonful soda. Bake twenty minutes.

---

*Custard.*—One pint milk, two eggs, one-half cup sugar, one-half cup flour, flavor and fill the cakes when cool.

Miss Carpenter.

---

*Almond Cake.*—Two cupfuls sugar, three-fourths of a cupful of butter, whites of five eggs, one cupful milk, three cupfuls flour, two teaspoonfuls baking powder, one teaspoonful of extract. Bake in layers and put together with the following custard : One cupful chopped almonds, one of sweet cream, two tablespoonfuls sugar, one tablespoonful cornstarch, one-half teaspoonful almond extract. Let the cream come to a boil, then add sugar, corn starch and almonds, and stir till it thickens. When cool, add extract and use between the layers, frosting the top.

Miss L. Dresher.

---

*White Cake.*—One cupful of butter beaten to a cream with two cupfuls of sugar and one of corn starch; add whites of eight eggs whipped stiff, a cupful of cold water and two cupfuls of flour, in which three teaspoonfuls of baking powder has been sifted very thoroughly, flavoring with vanilla. This will make seven layers, baked in a nine-inch tin. For the icing between the layers, beat two whites of eggs with two cupfuls confectioner's sugar, add juice of one lemon and two teaspoonfuls vanilla.

H. N. A.

---

*Ribbon Cake.*—Two and one-half cupfuls of sugur, one cupful each of butter and sweet milk, four cupfuls of flour, four eggs, two teaspoonfuls baking powder. Put one-third of the above in two long shallow tins. To the remainder add one cupful each of currants, raisins and citron, one teaspoonful each of cinnamon, allspice, cloves and nutmeg, and bake in one tin. Put the dark cake between the white layers, with frosting.

Mrs. C. H. Cleveland.

---

*Banana Cake.*—Cream three tablespoonfuls butter with two cupfuls of sugar, then add yolks of five eggs, well beaten, one cupful cold water, juice of one lemon, with grated peel, then three cupfuls of flour, into which have been sifted two tablesponfuls baking powder, and, lastly, the whites of three eggs. Bake in jelly tins. Filling: Beat together the whites of two eggs and one cupful powdered sugar, spread this on each layer and cover with the very thin slices of banana, placed closely, sprinkling each layer with juice and grated rind of a lemon. Ice the top of the cake.

Mrs. Marvin.

---

*Shrewsberry Cake.*—One coffeecupful of butter, one of sugar, one-half cnpful milk, two cupfuls of flour, three eggs, two teaspoonfuls baking powder, flavor with lemon. Drop one large spoonful of the dough into buttered cups and bake in a quick oven.

Miss Bartges.

---

*Chocolate Cake.*—One-half cupful butter, two cupfuls of sugar, three of flour, four eggs, two teaspoonfuls baking powder. Bake in jelly tins. Put the layers together with one cupful chocolate grated, one scant cupful of milk, one cupful of sugar, boiled till it threads from spoon. Just at the last add a small piece of butter.

Miss Josie A. Kent.

---

*Orange Cake.*—One cupful of butter, two of sugar, three and one-fourth cupfuls of flour, one cupful of milk, yolks of five eggs, whites of two, one and one-half teaspoonfuls baking powder, juice of one orange. Bake in jelly tins. Spread between the layers an icing made of white of three eggs, beaten stiff with sugar, juice of one and grated rind of two orages.

Mrs. E. A. Wilson.

---

*Silver Cake.*—Two cupfuls of sugar, one cupful of butter, one cupful of milk, four cupfuls of flour, one teaspoonful cream tartar, one-half teaspoonful soda, whites of five eggs.

Mrs. Alden,

---

*Gold Frosting.*—The yolk of one egg to nine heaping teaspoonfuls of pulverized sugar, flavor with vanilla. Use the day it is made.

Mrs. J. J. Harter.

---

*Cheap Fruit Cake.*—One cup butter, one cup sugar, one cup molasses, one cup of sweet milk, three cups of flour, four eggs, two teaspoonfuls baking powder, two pounds finely chopped raisins, one nutmeg. This will make two good sized loaves.

Mrs. Marvin.

---

*Cookies.*—Beat together two-thirds of a cup butter, one cup sugar, and two well beaten eggs, three tablespoonfuls milk, two teaspoonfuls baking powder, sifted into the flour, mix soft as can be rolled, and bake in a quick oven.

*Cream Cake.*—Four eggs, one cup sugar, one of flour, two teaspoonfuls baking powder, one tablespoonful of milk. Bake in three layers.

*Filling.*—One pint sweet cream, whipped stiff, mixed with one teacup of sugar. Miss McClure.

*Corn Starch Cake.*—One coffeecup of sugar, one-half cup butter, creamed thoroughly together; add one-half cup milk, one-half cup each of flour and corn starch, two teaspoonfuls baking powder, white of five eggs, whipped stiff; flavor to taste.

Miss McClure.

*Sponge Cake.*—Beat separately yolks and white of four eggs, put them together, add one cup sugar, which must be beaten well with the eggs, one cup of flour, three tablespoonfuls cold water, two teaspoonfuls baking powder, flavoring to taste.

Mrs. J. H. Collins.

*White Mountain Cake.*—Beat to a cream one-half cup of butter and one and one-half cups sugar, add one-half cup corn starch, then one-half cup of milk, in which one-half teaspoonful of soda has been dissolved, then one and one-half cups of flour, in which has been sifted one teaspoonful of cream tartar, lastly, the well beaten whites of six eggs. Mrs. Alden.

*Sand Tarts.*—Twelve ounces of butter, one pound sugar, two pounds flour, one egg, two tablespoonfuls cold water. Roll thin, cut in squares; wash the top with white of egg, sprinkle with cinnamon and loaf sugar, equal parts, and put blanched almonds on the top and bake. Mrs. Ganter.

*Sugar Cookies.*—One cup butter, two cups sugar, three eggs, three-fourths teaspoonful soda, wet with one tablespoonful boiling water, flour to roll soft. May Burlison.

*Nut Cookies.*—One cup butter, two cups sugar, one-half cup cold water, yolks four eggs, three teaspoonfuls baking powder, one cup chopped nuts, flour to roll stiff. H. N. Angel.

*Cookies.*—One cup sugar, two-thirds of a cup butter, same quantity sweet milk, one egg, two teaspoonfuls baking powder. Knead soft, roll thin, and bake in a quick oven. Lena Wright.

*Fritters.*—Ten tablespoonfuls melted butter, as many of sugar, three eggs. Mix stiff, cut in squares, make six or eight incisions in each square, lift by taking each alternate strip with thumb and finger. Fry in hot lard. A. H.

*Cocoanut Cookies.*—Two cups sugar, one of butter, one teaspoonful soda, dissolved in a tablespoonful of milk, one cocoanut, and flour sufficient to roll. Mrs. J. J. Harter.

---

*Cookies.*—Three-fourths cup butter, one cup coffee, sugar, two eggs, two tablespoonfuls milk, one teaspoonful vanilla, two teaspoonfuls baking powder, flour to roll out thin. Spread with jelly put two together with jelly between, and bake in a quick ovan.

Mrs. W. B. Raymond.

---

*Sugar Cookies.*—One quart flour, two cups sugar, one of them white, one brown, one half cup butter, same quantity of milk, two teaspoonfuls baking powder. Stir yolks of eggs with butter, then add other ingredients, flavering to taste.

Miss Bartges.

---

*Almond Jumbles.*—One pound butter, one pound sugar, one and three-fourths pounds flour, one-half pound almonds, in the shell, whites four eggs, yolks of six. Cream the butter and sugar, add eggs, beaten separately, then flour. Use mace or nutmeg as flavoring. Work as little as possible, roll thin. Wash the top of the cakes with white of egg, place on them strips of almond, blanched, sprinkle with sugar and cinnamon and bake.

Mrs. Raff.

---

*Cookies.*—Cream together one-half cup butter and one and one-fourth cups sugar, add four tablespoonfuls thick cream, whites four eggs, yolks of three, three full cups flour, with one heaping teaspoonful baking powder thoroughly sifted in flour, stir as for any cake, and use one teaspoonful of dough for each cookie. Mrs. W. C. Jacobs

---

*Cookies.*—One cup of butter, two cups of sugar, one-half cup of milk, one egg, one-half teaspoonful soda, flour to roll.

Mrs. Alden.

---

*Ginger Snaps.*—Put at once into two quarts of flour, (it will seem too much,) one cup butter and lard mixed, one cup of molasses, one of very brown sugar, one egg, unbeaten, one tablespoonful soda stirred into the molasses, one tablespoonful of ginger, same quantity of mixed spices, teaspoonful of salt. Knead half an hour, adding flour as needed. There is no danger of too much flour. Bake in a quick oven. This measure will make one hundred snaps. H. N. A.

---

*Ginger Snaps.*—One cup butter, one of sugar, one of molasses, one tablespoonful ginger, same quantity of cloves, one teaspoonful of soda. Flora Sumner.

*Molasses Pound Cake.*—One cup each of butter, sugar, and milk, in which last dissolve one teaspoonful of soda, two cups molasses, five eggs, five cups of flour. Beat together butter and sugar, then add other ingredients, spicing with cinnamon and nutmeg. Mrs. R. H. Wright.

---

*Hard Ginger-bread.*—One and one-half cups molasses, one cup sour milk, one-half cup of butter, one tablespoonful each, of ginger and soda, made into a stiff dough, roll moderately thin, and spread in pans. Mrs. Howard.

---

*Raised Doughnuts.*—Four large cups of bread dough, one large cup of butter, two even cups sugar, four eggs, one teaspoonful soda, one tablespoonful cinnamon, one nutmeg. Let this, well beaten together, rise over night, in the morning roll out, let them rise again, then fry. Mrs. M. Sumner.

---

*Old-fashioned Plain Doughnuts.*—Three cups bread sponge, one tablespoonful lard, one tablespoonful of sugar, mixed in with the hands. Add flour, till the dough can be handled, but keep as soft as possible, mold and let it rise. When light, turn out on the board, cut into strips, without molding again, twist and fry in "still hot" lard. Mrs. Latham.

---

*Doughnuts.*—One-half teacup butter, one of sugar, and three eggs beaten together, two cups sour milk, one teaspoonful soda, (or two cups sweet milk, and three teaspoonfuls baking powder,) flour to make a soft dough. Let them stand an hour before frying. Mrs. J. H. Collins.

---

*Snow Balls.*—Beat well together one cup sugar, one egg, and four tablespoonfuls of melted lard, add one teacup of milk, (in cold weather warm the milk,) and mix as stiff as can be stirred with flour into which two teaspoonfuls of baking powder have been stirred; let it stand fifteen minutes, then knead as soft as can be handled; cut into inch and a half squares and fry. When thoroughly cold, roll in pulverized sugar. Miss McClure.

---

*Boiled Frosting.*—Boil one teacup of sugar in an iron spoonful of water; when waxy, pour slowly into the white of one egg, beaten stiff, stirring constantly till thick. Miss King.

---

*Fried Cakes.*—Seven tablespoonfuls of lard, one cup sweet milk, same of sugar, two eggs, two teaspoonfuls baking powder, salt and nutmeg. Sara Buckingham.

---

*Gateau a la Fortin.*—Two cupfuls of "Cerealine;" four cupfuls of flour, one cupful of butter, two cupfuls of sugar, four eggs one teaspoonful of baking powder, two cupfuls of seeded raisins, one and one-half cupfuls of milk, one teaspoonful of extract of almonds and vanilla, mixed. Rub the butter, sugar, and eggs very smooth; add the flour and baking powder sifted together, then add the "Cerealine," raisins, milk, and extracts; mix into medium batter and bake in a cake mould, in a quick, steady oven.

---

*Doughnuts.*—One egg, one cup milk, one cup sugar, two teaspoonfuls melted butter, three heaping teaspoonfuls baking powder, flour to mold. Mrs. Blackie.

---

*Sand Tarts.*—One cup butter, one and one-half cups sugar, two well beaten eggs, half teaspoonful soda, three teaspoonfuls water, flour to make them stiff enough to roll out thin. Baste the top with the white of an egg and sprinkle sugar on them, after cutting them out like cookies. Mrs. Humphrey.

---

*Cookies.*—One cup of butter, two of sugar, four eggs, one teaspoon of soda dissolved in two teaspoons of milk, flour to roll out thin, three teaspoons carraway seeds. Will keep a long time.

Mrs. Humphrey.

---

*Ginger Sponge Cakes.*— One pint molasses, two eggs, one tablespoon soda, six ounces butter, one teaspoon ginger, one cup water. Drop from a spoon after flour enough has been added to do so, on buttered ~~toast~~. C. P. H.

*Prize Fotograf Cake.*—To produce this delightful cake in the highest degree of perfection, great care must be observed at every step. The purest ingredients, the most exact proportions, the cleanest of dishes and hands are necessary. There are various designs in which to form these Cakes, Medallions, Cups, etc., being the most usual. There are various grades, also, as the Silver Cake, the Gold Cake, the Bronze Cake, etc. By way of encouraging greater skill and perfection in the art and science most useful to labor and commercial progress—in which cake baking is included—prizes have been offered for the highest degree of excellence. The great State of Ohio, the United States of America, and all the countries of the world combined, have offered prizes for superiority. In the art of Photography, James F. Ryder, of 239 Superior Street, Cleveland, Ohio, has been awarded FOURTEEN GRAND PRIZES from State, Nation, and World for superiority. Hence, RYDER TAKES THE CAKE.

THE FOTOGRAF CAKE.

# THE LEGEND OF CEREALINE.

"'Twas the women who in Autumn
Stripped the yellow husks of harvest,
Stripped the garments from Mondamin,
Even as Hiawatha taught them."

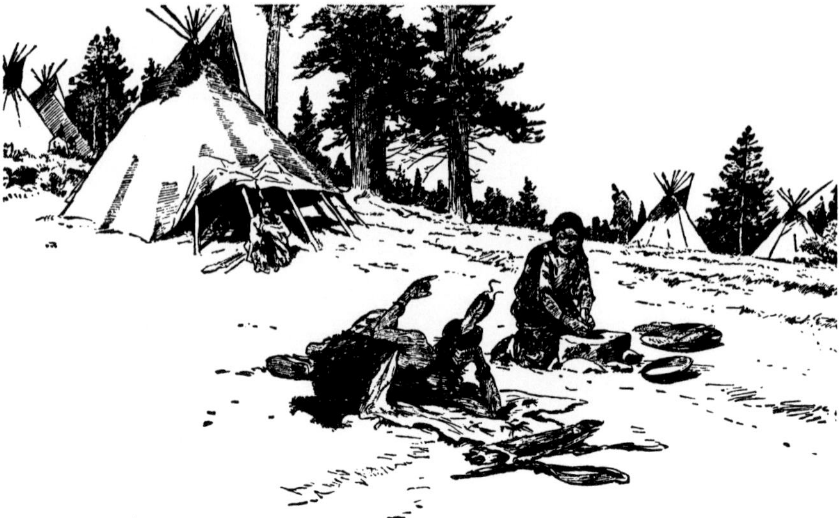

To the lovely Minnehaha,
Hiawatha spake in this wise:
"Tell me of the Food so wondrous,
Of this Cerealine you prize so;
Tell the secrets of the Cook Book."
Minnehaha answered, smiling,
As she mixed the creamy batter:
"O my husband, 'tis a marvel,
And a food of countless virtues.
Lo, it yields us waffles, muffins,
Yields us griddle-cakes and puddings;
Good to lighten bread and pie-crust,
Twice as nourishing as oatmeal,
Thrice as nutritive as buckwheat,
More nutritious far than rice is,
Excellent for soup and porridge,
Far surpassing maccaroni,
Noodles, vermicelli, sago;
Good for breakfast, dinner, supper,
Good for strong men or the weakly,
Good for women and papooses."
"'Tis a blessing to us old folks,"
Called Nakomis from the wigwam.

**The series of twelve original pictures, illustrating "Hiawatha's Fasting," of which the above is a small example, will be mailed to any one who will mention where this advertisement was seen and enclose a two-cent stamp for postage to the Cerealine Mfg. Co., Columbus, Indiana.**

# CONFECTIONS.

CANDIES.—"Sweet are thy sticks and sticky are thy sweets."

*Lemon Ice.*--One pound white sugar, juice of thee or four lemons, one quart of water. Pare the lemons as thin as possible in order to cut through the little oil vessels. Heat a little of the water and pour it over the rinds, allowing it to stand long enough to extract the flavor. Stir into the mixture the whites of two eggs, slightly beaten just as it is put into the freezer. To make *nectar ice* add to the above very little vanilla, and a little currant juice, which last gives a delicate pink color. To make an ice hard it is necessary, after it has been stirred until frozen, to remove the paddle, take out the packing, repack from the foundation, and let the ice stand one or two hours in the new packing, before using.

Mrs. E. D. Dodge.

---

*Butter Scotch.*—Three tablespoons molasses, two tablespoons sugar, two tablespoons water, one tablespoon butter, boil until it becomes as soft as wax.

---

*Another.*—Two cups brown sugar, half cup water, one teaspoon vinegar butter the size of an egg. Mrs. Humphrey.

---

"*No Egg*" *Ice Cream.*—Boil together one-half cup of flour and one pint of milk, twenty minutes; add three pints cold milk, sugar, flavor to taste, and freeze.

---

*Ice Cream.*—One pint sweet cream, same quantity new milk, two teaspoonfuls arrowroot, one-half pound sugar, yolks five eggs. Place the milk on the stove, heat it and stir in the arrowroot, wet in cold milk. Pour this on the yolks and sugar, well beaten together, and cook till as thick as boiled custard. When cool, flavor with one teaspoonful vanilla, or cook one-half a vanilla bean in the milk, and add cream well whipped. Freeze, stirring for fifteen minutes, then take out the dasher and let stand for two hours. Mrs. W. B. Raymond.

---

*Coffee Ice.*—Freeze one-half pint strongest coffee, same quantity rich cream, and one-fourth pound sugar, well stirred together.

*Wine Jelly.*—Soak one box gelatine in one quart cold water for two or three hours. Then add three pints boiling water, grate in rind of four lemons, also use juice of the lemons, one pint wine, one pint sugar, stir well and strain into a mold, and set on ice to harden. Mrs. A. J. M.

---

*French Cream.*—Break into a glass the whites of one egg or more, add an equal quantity of cold water, and stir in confectioner's sugar, (XXX,) until stiff enough to mold into shape with the fingers. Flavor to taste. To one egg I use one teaspoonful of extract one-third each of lemon, vanilla and orange. Vanilla or lemon alone is fine. These creams are better the day after making them. Mrs. J. A. Mason.

---

*Fruit Candy.*—One cocoanut. Wet with milk of the cocoanut one and one-half pounds of white sugar; put it into a saucepan and let it heat slowly, then boil rapidly five minutes, add the cocoanut, finely grated, and boil ten minutes longer, stirring constantly. Try a little on a cool plate, and if it forms a fine paste when cool, remove it from the fire. Pour a part of it out in a large tin, lined with buttered paper; then add to the remainder, one-fourth pound stoned raisins, one-half pound blanched almonds, one pint pecans, and one-half cup chopped walnuts. Pour the mixture over the candy in the pan, and when cold cut in squares. Mrs. E. O. Stanley.

---

*Kisses.*—Beat for an hour one pint pulverized sugar, whites eight eggs, one tablespoonful cornstarch. About five minutes before the beating is finished, add one small teaspoonful cream tartar, and bake on buttered paper twenty minutes.

Mrs. W. B. Raymond.

---

*Fruit Jelly.*—Soak one-half box of gelatine in half a pint of cold water an hour, add juice of two lemons, and three oranges, two cups white sugar, and over the whole pour one-half pint of boiling water. Fill a mold half full of pieces of fruit, any kinds. If bananas, grapes and oranges are used, slice six bananas a quarter of an inch thick, divide four oranges into sections, cutting into two pieces, put one-fourth pound white grapes in whole, pour over all the gelatine mixture, set on the ice to harden.

Mrs. Dodge.

---

*Strawberry Ice.*—Crush two quarts of strawberries, with two pounds sugar. Let them stand an hour or more, then squeeze through a straining cloth, pressing out all the juice. Add to this an equal quantity of water, and when half frozen, the beaten whites of eggs, in the proportion of three eggs to each quart of syrup.

Mrs. Dodge.

*Raspberry Vinegar*.—Put six quarts red raspberries and three quarts currants into a stone jar and cover with vinegar. Stir every day for nine days, strain through a double cloth, and add to each pint of juice one pound of sugar. Boil twenty-five minutes bottle but not seal. This will make eight quarts vinegar.

Mrs. W. B. Raymond.

---

*Butter Scotch*.—Boil till it hardens on a spoon, two cups sugar, two tablespoonfuls water, a piece of butter size of an egg, without stirring, then pour in buttered pans to cool.

---

*Roasted Almonds*.—Shell and blanch the almonds, put them into a saucepan with some salt, set them into the oven till they are hot. Remove them from the oven, add to the almonds a small piece of butter and shake over the fire till browned, taking care that they do not burn. Mrs. J. A. Mason.

---

*Kisses*.—Beat to a stiff froth the whites of four eggs, and half a pound of powdered sugar, (the more thoroughly these are beaten, the stiffer are the kisses.) Bake on wet paper, laid on hard wood boards in a moderate oven.

---

*Hickory Nut Maccaroons*.—Mix together one pound powdered sugar, one pound finely chopped nuts, one tablespoonful of flour two small teaspoonfuls baking powder, and unbeaten whites of five eggs, and drop from a teaspoon upon buttered paper, in baking tins. Do not put too near each other, bake a light brown in a moderate oven. Weigh the nuts in the shell.

---

*Hickory Nut Maccaroons*.—Whites of three eggs beaten stiff, add one pint of sugar, a bowl of hickory nut meats chopped very fine and into which has been mixed half a cup of flour. Bake in a moderate oven. These are excellent, if butternuts be used instead of hickory nuts. Mrs. F. S. N.

---

*Maccaroons*.—One pound of almonds, blanched and pounded, whites of three eggs well beaten, one pound pulverized sugar, sifted, mix well together and drop into little cakes on buttered paper, dredge them with a little sugar and bake.

---

*Chocalate Carmels*.—Boil together one cupful each of grated chocalate, milk, molasses and sugar, with butter size of an egg, until it will harden when dropped into cold water, flavor with vanilla, pour on buttered tins and when pretty cool mark off into squares.

---

*Jellied Fruit*.—The juice of two lemons and two oranges, one-half box gelatine, in half a cupful cold water, add half a cupful boiling water, one and one-half cupfuls sugar. Slice four bananas and strip two oranges, mix with the jelly and set in a cool place. Mrs. N. P. Goodhue.

---

*Jellied Fruit.*—Soak a half box of gelatine in a cupful and a half of warm water; when the gelatine is dissolved add a cupful of sugar, the juice of two lemons and one orange, and one and a half cupfuls of boiling water, strain into a mold which has been half filled with sliced bananas and quartered oranges and set on the ice till ready to serve. Mrs. E. O. Stanley.

---

*Tutti Frutti.*—Put one pint of brandy into a jar; begin with the first fruits of the season, putting each variety into the jar with as much sugar as fruit, cutting pine apples, peaches and large fruits into small bits; add fruit and sugar as long as the fruit season lasts, also add pounded nut meats, cork tightly and put away to use. It is very rich and to be served daintily with ice cream, charlotte, fusse, etc., for desserts. Miss Carpenter.

---

*Russian Cream.*—One cupful white sugar, one quart milk, three eggs, beaten separately, one-half box gelatine; beat the sugar with the yolks of the eggs, dissolve the gelatine in one-half pint of warm water, which when dissolved is added to the boiling milk, also eggs and sugar, stirring as for custard, flavor and add whites of eggs, While hot, pour into molds and serve cold.

Miss Carpenter.

---

*French Cream Candy.*—Two cupfuls granulated sugar, one of cold water, one and one-half table spoonfuls arrowroot. Dissolve the arrowroot in a little of the water and pour over the sugar. Boil from ten to twenty minutes, stirring constantly. When the syrup thickens and drops rather heavily from the spoon, take from the fire and set the sauce pan in a pan of cold water and beat into a smooth white cream. Before it is cold flavor and mold into any desired shape. If it crumbles it has boiled too long; add a little water and boil again; if sticky it has not boiled long enough. By using dates, nuts, etc., quite a variety can be made. Miss Perkins.

---

*Almond Maccaroons.*—Prepare the almonds the day before you wish to use them, by blanching them, (putting them into hot water and rubbing off the skins,) and when perfectly cold, pounding them as fine as possible, adding to each pound of almonds one tablespoonful of rosewater, and a little extract of almond to make a smooth paste. Cover closely and set away in a cool place until the next day. Then to every pound of nuts made into this paste, allow one pound of granulated sugar, the beaten whites of eight eggs, and one teaspoonful of nutmeg.

Stir the sugar and whites of egg lightly together then whip in gradually the almond paste. Drop on buttered white paper, laid in baking dish, spoonfuls of the mixture far enough apart that they will not run together. Sift powdered sugar over them and bake in a quick oven to a delicate brown. If, when dropping them, they run into irregular shapes, add more sugar.

Mrs. F. S. Newton.

---

*Cream of Nectar, or Home Soda.*—One gallon water, four pounds sugar, six ounces tartaric acid, two ounces cream tartar, one ounce epsom salts, whites of six eggs well beaten in a pint of water. Thicken with two spoonfuls wheat flour, and put all together in a kettle and skim before boiling. When cool, flavor. Put into two-thirds of a tumbler of water two tablespoonfuls of this mixture, add one-fourth teaspoonful soda, stir till it foams and drink.

Mrs. E. S. Day.

# K. GINTZ

Can Guarantee you Great Bargains in Parlor, Chamber and Dining Room

# FURNITURE,

Matresses, &c. ☞ Repairing a Specialty.

**176 South Howard St., AKRON, OHIO.**

---

**Housekeepers will always Find Bargains and Save Money at**

# FRANK'S BAZAAR,

**136 South Howard Street, Phœnix Block,**

**AKRON, OHIO.**

---

**FURNACES, FURNACES, FURNACES,**

# FURNACES!

**FURNACES, FURNACES, FURNACES,**

THE BEST AT

## JAHANT & WEBER'S.

**If you contemplate buying one, call on them before you buy.**

---

**FOR LADIES', MISSES' AND CHILDREN'S**

# FINE SHOES,

**IN ALL STYLES AND LOW PRICES, CALL ON**

# STEESE & GOOD,

THE ONE PRICE SHOE HOUSE, *145 South Howard Street,*

**AKRON, OHIO.**

# PICKLES.

*Spanish Pickles.*—Six dozen large green cucumbers, twelve large green peppers, one peck of onions, one peck of green tomatoes cut in slices, sprinkle through them one quart of salt, let them stand all night, in the morning drain them well, then add two ounces of mustard seed, two ounces of mace, two ounces pepper, two ounces of cloves, two ounces of celery seed, two ounces of turmeric, three tablespoonfuls of ground mustard, one pint of g ated horse-radish, one pound of brown sugar. Cover this with vinegar, let it boil one hour.

---

*Pickled Peppers.*—Cut stems out in a circle and preserve them, fill each pepper with a mixture of fine chopped cabbage, horse-radish, mustard-seed and salt. Replace the pieces cut out, and tie with coarse thread, pack in stone jars, and fill the jars with cold, sharp vinegar, ready for use in two weeks.

---

*Pickled Cucumbers.*—Having washed the cucumbers, lay them in a crock with alternate layers of salt, and let them remain twenty-four hours, then rinse in cold water, pack in jars in alternate layers of cucumbers, and of spices and red pepper. Cover with vinegar, sugar to taste, scald and seal. Mrs. C. A. Collins.

---

*Pickled Onions.*—Take small white onions, put them over the fire in cold water, with a handful of salt. When the water becomes scalding hot, take out and peel off skins, dry and put in a jar. Boil half an ounce each allspice and cloves in a quart of vinegar, take out spice and pour vinegar over onions while hot. Tie up jar when vinegar is cold, and keep in a dry place.

---

*Spiced Grapes or Currants.*—Boil and strain through a colander to remove skins and seeds. To six pounds of grapes add three pounds of sugar, one pint of vinegar two tablespoons of cinnamon, one tablespoon each of cloves and mace. Boil one hour.

---

*Mixed Pickles.*—Three hundred very small cucumbers, eight large green peppers, sliced, one large root of horseradish, two quarts small white onions, one head cauliflower, all put into a brine made of ice water, strong enough to bear up an egg, where they must remain twenty-four hours. Drain three hours and pour over the pickles two gallons white wine vinegar, scalded with one-fourth pound white, and same quantity of black mustard seed, one teaspoonful cayenne pepper and one ounce of turmeric. When cold add one pint mustard, prepared as for table.

Mrs. C. Johnston.

---

*Chili Sauce.*—Twenty-four large ripe tomatoes, two red peppers, eight tablespoonfuls sugar, four tablespoonfuls salt, six cupfuls of vinegar, two tablespoonfuls each of ginger, cinnamon, cloves, nutmeg; chop all very fine, boil until quite thick, and bottle. Mrs. Blackie.

---

*Mixed Pickles.*—One peck of small onions, two hundred small cucumbers, two heads of cauliflower, three large green peppers, twelve small red peppers, one quart green or lima beans. five quarts vinegar, one and one-half pounds mustard. Heat three quarts vinegar, mix smooth the mustard in two quarts, then add to the heated vinegar; when thick as cream, turn on pickles, having laid all but the peppers in salt for twenty-four hours previously. This makes four gallons. Mrs. F. A. Fauver.

# COOKERY FOR THE SICK.

*Raw Egg.*—Beat a fresh egg very light, sweeten to taste, pour into a glass with two tablespoonfuls of port wine, beat again and drink.

*Mulled Jelly.*—Beat with one tablespoonful of currant or grape jelly, the white of one egg and a little loaf sugar, pour over it a half pint of boiling water and break into it a stick of dry toast or a craker.

*Mulled Buttermilk.*—Heat in a saucepan a pint of fresh buttermilk, add a little salt and cook a tablespoon heaping full of corn meal in the milk ten minutes.

*Beef Tea.*—Cut tender, juicy beef into very small pieces, put into a strong bottle, cork tightly, place in a kettle of cold water, bring to a boil and boil two hours.

*Panada.*—Put some very thin parts of light bread into a bowl, grate over this some nutmeg, pour over boiling water, cover and let it stand a few minutes.

*Arrowroot Custard.*—While a pint of milk is boiling, stir into it a large spoonful of arrowroot, mixed smooth with a little cold milk. Let it boil three minutes and when cool add two well beaten eggs, sugar and nutmeg to taste. Place where it will be scalding hot, stirring constantly, and as soon as it boils turn into a mold.

*Cream of Cerealine.* Into two quarts of veal or chicken stock stir two cupfuls of "Cerealine;" boil for ten minutes; season with salt and pepper; rub through a sieve; return all to a soup kettle; add one cupful of milk, and bring it to a boil again; beat the yolks of two eggs very lightly, and put into a tureen ; pour over them one cupful of boiling cream ; stir well together and follow with the hot soup, and serve with croutons or fried bread.

*Gruel.*—Take one pint of boiling water; stir into it "Cerealine," a tablespoonful at a time, at intervals, keeping the mixture constantly stirred until the desired consistency is obtained, season with salt and a little butter, to suit the taste, and let it simmer for about five minutes.

*Toast Water.*—Toast stale bread until quite brown, being very careful not to burn it. Put it into a large bowl, pour over it boiling water and cover closely. A bit of ice put into the tumbler when given to drink is an improvement.

*Corn Coffee.*—Grind parched corn, pour on boiling water, a pint of water to a spoonful of corn, boil three minutes. Season to taste.

*Cough Syrup.*—Stew an ounce of licorice root, till the strength is extracted, and in the tea dissolve one ounee gum arabic. Dose, a teaspoonful often.

*Flaxseed Lemonade.*—Stir four tablespoonfuls of flaxseed into a quart of boiling water, and keep it just below the boiling point four hou s, when it should be reduced to a pint, strain, squeeze into it the juice of a large lemon, adding sugar to make it palateable. One tablespoonful every half hour. Miss A. J.

# SCRAPS.

*Scraps.*—English manufacturers are careful to give explicit directions, for the washing of hose of black, blue, and other plain colors. The manner of setting the color is simple. Before wearing the hose, make a strong soap suds with warm water; in which wash thoroughly the stockings on the wrong side. Rinse them in clear warm, water, then in clear cold water.

---

*To Remove Rust From Steel.*—Cover the steel with sweet oil well rubbed on it, and lay aside for forty-eight hours. Then rub with unslaked lime till the rust has disappeared.

---

*To Remove Machine Oil.*—Wash with cold water and soap, hot water sets the stain.

---

*To Prevent Calicos From Fading.*—Make a strong solution of salt, allowing half a pint of salt to a quart of water. Put the material into this while hot, let it lie for a time, then take out and wash as usual. This is equally good for linens, and percales.

---

*Camphor Ice.*—Two ounces spermaceti, three ounces best olive oil, one ounce white wax, camphor gum the size of a hickory nut. Melt and stir until white. Mrs. Humphrey.

---

*To Remove Mildew.*—Rub soft soap on the spots and expose to the sun, repeating two or three times.

---

*Red Ants.*—Having washed and wiped thoroughly the cupboard, sprinkle in salt rubbing well into cracks and crevices. This properly done will so annoy the pests that they will leave

---

*Scraps.*—If a person begins to grate a nutmeg at the stalk end, it will prove hollow throughout, whereas the same nutmeg grated at the other end would have proved sound and solid to the last.

Do not pour boiling water on trays as it will make them crack and peel off, but have a sponge wet with warm water and a little soap if the tray be very dirty. then rub with a cloth.

A very simple way to cool liquids is to wrap a moistened cloth around the bottle and expose to the rays of the sun, this will have the desired effect.

A few drops of any perfumed oil will secure libraries from the consuming effects of mould and damp. Mrs. Humphrey.

*Scraps.*—A basin of water placed in the oven while meat is roasting, will prevent its burning.

Never put salt on steak while cooking, as salt extracts the juices and they are lost.

Any quantity of oil can be removed from a carpet or any woolen stuff by applying plentifully and faithfully, buckwheat, flour or corn meal.

Put a piece of unslaked lime into a bottle of water, set it in a cool dark place and keep corked. It will be ready at any time. A little put into milk or cream will prevent its turning, and will not affect the taste unpleasantly. It is also excellent to cleanse bottles or jugs which have had milk in them. Some add a little to the bread sponge to insure sweetness.

A piece of horse radish placed in a jar with pickles will prevent the rising of scum.

A mixture of common clay and benzine will clean marble.

Gilt frames may be cleaned by first dusting, then washing with the mixture of three ounces of whites of eggs and one ounce of soda, applying with a soft cloth.

To check bleeding from nose or cuts, make rolls of cobweb, insert or bind on.

If your coal fire is low, a tablespoonful of salt thrown on will make it blaze finely.

In boiling meat for soup, put the meat into cold water, to extract the juices; if for cooking the meat for itself, put the meat into hot water, as thus a crust is formed at once by which the juices are retained in the meat.

---

*For Cleaning Clothing or Carpets.*—One fourth pound castile soap, same quantity of ammonia, one pound ether, one pound of glycerine, and one pound of spirits of wine. Cut the soap fine and beat in a quart of soft water, until entirely dissolved; then add with other ingredients, four quarts of water. Mrs. Howard.

---

*Hair Wash.*—Powder fine and dissolve in one quart of hot water, one ounce of borax and half an ounce of camphor gum. Dampen the hair often with the fluid, which not only cleanses but strengthens the hair.

---

*Cure for Hams.*—Make brine strong enough to bear an egg; then for every one hundred pounds of meat add one fourth pound saltpeter, dissolved, and three quarts of molasses, stir well and pour over the meat when cold. After standing in this brine four weeks they will be ready for smoking. Mrs. H. H. Brown.

---

*Baking Powder.*—Sift together seven times, seven ounces best baking soda and sixteen ounces pure cream tartar. Keep in tight boxes. H. N. Angel.

*Corned Beef.*—For every one hundred pounds of meat use six pounds fine salt, six gallons water, one-fourth pound saltpeter, same quantity of soda, two quarts molasses, scald together and skim. Pack the meat closely in a barrel and pour brine over it hot.

Mrs. H. H. Brown.

---

*Baking Powder.*—One-fourth pound of baking soda, one-half pound of cream tartar, one-half package corn starch. Dry in a moderate oven for one hour, the soda and cream tartar; sift three times, add corn starch and sift three times again. Keep in tight boxes.

---

*Fruit Spots.*—Fruit spots may be removed by pouring boiling water over them before washing. Tea or coffee stains may be removed by the same method.

## ANTIDOTES FOR POISONS.

*Acids.*—Magnesia, soda, or soap dissolved in water.

*Alkali.*—Vinegar or any acid.

*Ammonia.*—Lemon juice, vinegar, or any acid.

*Alcohol.*—After an emetic, dash cold water on the head and give soda.

*Arsenic.*—Whites of eggs, chalk and water or lime water.

*Laudanum.*—Coffee, acids, and cold water on the head, with friction.

*Belladonna.*—Emetics, then acids, as lemonade, vinegar, etc.

*Morphine.*—Same as for laudanum

*Charcoal.*—Take the patient into the fresh air, dash water on the head, stimulate lungs and nostrils with ammonia, rub the chest vigorously.

*Corrosive Sublimate.*—White of eggs, flour and water, salt and water.

*Creosote.*—Whites of eggs and emetics.

*Lead.*—Alum and cathartics.

*Mushrooms.*—Emetics, and plenty of vinegar with doses of ether.

*Nitrate of Silver.*—Common salt then emetics.

*Opium.*—Same as for laudanum

*Nux Vomica.*—First emetics then brandy.

*Oxalic Acid.*—Any alkali, as soda.

*Prussic Acid*—Soda, hot brandy and water with turpentine.

*Snake Bite.*—Strong hartshorn outside and in, sweet oil and stimulants, and having applied a ligature above the part bitten apply a cupping glass, or suck out the poison, being careful not to swallow.

*Tartar Emetic.*—Large doses of nut galls, Peruvian, or white oak bark.

*Verdigris.*—Large doses of whites of eggs in water.

*White Vitriol.*—Large doses of milk.

## TABLE OF WEIGHTS AND MEASURES.

One quart sifted flour weighs a pound.
One quart sifted Indian meal weighs one pound and one ounce.
One pint soft butter, well packed weighs a pound.
One and one third pints powdered sugar weigh a pound.
Two coffee cups powdered sugar, level full weigh a pound.
One pint of granulated sugar, heaped, weighs fourteen ounces.
Two teacups, level full weigh a pound.
One pint brown sugar is thirteen ounces.
One tablespoonful butter weighs an ounce.
One pint sugar is a pound.
Two cups butter are a pound.

| | Time for Boiling. Minutes. | Sugar to qt. Ounces. |
|---|---|---|
| Raspberries | 6 | 4 |
| Blackberries | 6 | 6 |
| Plums | 10 | 10 |
| Pears | 20 | 6 |
| Peaches | 15 | 4 |
| Crab Apples | 25 | 4 |
| Ripe Currants | 6 | 8 |
| Grapes | 10 | 8 |

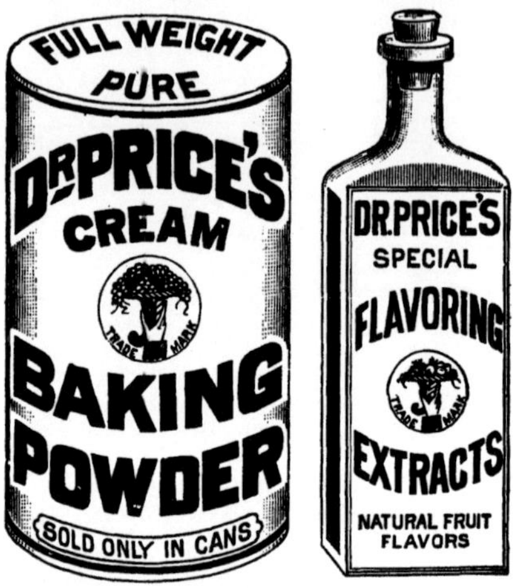
FULL WEIGHT
PURE
DR PRICE'S
CREAM
TRADE MARK
BAKING
POWDER
SOLD ONLY IN CANS
DR. PRICE'S
SPECIAL
FLAVORING
TRADE MARK
EXTRACTS
NATURAL FRUIT
FLAVORS